Urinary Incontinence in Adults: Acute and Chronic Management

Urinary Incontinence in Adults Guideline Update Panel

J. Andrew Fantl, MD (Co-Chair)
Diane Kaschak Newman, RNC, MSN, FAAN (Co-Chair)
Joyce Colling, PhD, RN, FAAN
John O.L. DeLancey, MD
Christopher Keeys, PharmD
Richard Loughery, FACHA
B. Joan McDowell, PhD, RN, FAAN
Peggy Norton, MD
Joseph Ouslander, MD
Jack Schnelle, PhD
David Staskin, MD
Jeannette Tries, MS, OTR
Vernon Urich, MD
Sharon H. Vitousek, MD
Barry D. Weiss, MD
Kristene Whitmore, MD

U.S. Department of Health and Human Services
Public Health Service
Agency for Health Care Policy and Research
Rockville, Maryland

AHCPR Publication No. 96-0682
March 1996

Guideline Development and Use

Guidelines are systematically developed statements to assist practitioner and patient decisions about appropriate health care for specific clinical conditions. This guideline update was developed by a private-sector panel convened by the Agency for Health Care Policy and Research (AHCPR). The panel employed an explicit, science-based methodology and expert clinical judgment to develop specific statements on patient assessment and management for the clinical condition selected.

Extensive literature searches were conducted and critical reviews and syntheses were used to evaluate empirical evidence and significant outcomes. Peer review and field review were undertaken to evaluate the validity, reliability, and utility of the guideline in clinical practice. The panel's recommendations are primarily based on the published scientific literature. When the scientific literature was incomplete or inconsistent in a particular area, the recommendations reflect the professional judgment of panel members and consultants.

Guideline updates are a result of a periodic review of the state of scientific information and technology. Updates reflect new research findings, experience, or technologies and provide specific recommendations in the field.

We believe that the AHCPR-assisted clinical practice guidelines will make positive contributions to the quality of care in the United States. We encourage practitioners and patients to use the information provided in this *Clinical Practice Guideline Update*. The recommendations may not be appropriate for use in all circumstances. Decisions to adopt any particular recommendation must be made by the practitioner in light of available resources and circumstances presented by individual patients.

Clifton R. Gaus, ScD
Administrator
Agency for Health Care Policy and Research

Publication of this guideline does not necessarily represent endorsement by the U.S. Department of Health and Human Services.

Abstract

Despite the prevalence of urinary incontinence (UI), the condition is widely underdiagnosed and underreported. Many health care providers remain uneducated about this condition, and individuals are often ashamed or embarrassed to seek professional help. Furthermore, UI diagnostic and treatment practices as well as associated medical costs vary widely. These factors prompted the selection of UI in adults as a topic for guideline development. A panel of experts used an extensive review of scientific literature as well as expert judgment and group consensus to develop this guideline. Findings and recommendations are presented for (1) prevention, identification, and evaluation of UI; (2) use of behavioral, pharmacologic, and surgical treatment as well as supportive devices; (3) long-term management of chronic intractable UI; and (4) education of health professionals and the public. The panel found evidence in the literature that the treatment of UI can improve or "cure" most patients. They concluded that all patients with UI should have a basic diagnostic evaluation and that behavioral and pharmacologic therapies are usually reasonable first steps in management. In addition, vigorous efforts should be made to educate the professional and lay public.

Acknowledgments

The panel wishes to acknowledge several other consultants and technical advisors. They have provided external reviews for the combined analyses, consultation during panel meetings, and testimony during the open forum. They are:

Consultants

Patricia Burns, PhD, RN, FAAN
Ananias Diokno, MD
Teh-Wei Hu, PhD

Donna Katzman McClish, PhD
Thelma Joan Wells, PhD, RN
Matthew Zack, MD, MPH

Technical Advisors

Jerry Blaivas, MD
Kari Bo, PE, PT, PhD
Carol Brink, MPH, RN
Linda Cardozo, MD
Alan Cottenden, PhD
Molly Dougherty, PhD, RN, FAAN
Sheila Fiers, RN, BSN, CETN
Cheryl Gartley
Katherine Jeter, EdD

Rhonda Kotarinos, MS, PT
Deborah Lekan-Rutledge, MSN, RN, C
Christine Norton, MA, RN
Mary H. Palmer, RNC, PhD, FAAN
Neil Resnick, MD
Carolyn Sampselle, PhD, RN, FAAN
Alan Wein, MD

Many other organizations and individuals also made significant contribution during the development of this guideline. Although they are too numerous to mention here, the Contributors section, which appears later in this document, lists individual consultants, peer reviewers, and support staff. Publication of this guideline would not have been possible without their collaborative efforts.

Contents

Foreword

Urinary incontinence (UI) affects approximately 13 million Americans in community and institutional settings. Despite its prevalence, and an estimated annual cost of more than $15 billion, most affected individuals do not seek help for incontinence, primarily because of embarrassment or because they are not aware that help is available. When individuals do seek help, evidence exists that practitioners are hesitant or ill prepared to discuss, diagnose, or treat the problem.

A number of Federal and private organizations have provided research funding for the study of UI. Data from these studies indicate that treatment of UI is effective in most people, but there is an increased need for efforts to inform and educate the public and health care providers about the condition. Furthermore, there are wide variations in the actual costs and methods of providing care for UI, in the actual costs per procedure, and the charges within each diagnostic group.

It is expected that UI will continue to be a significant health care problem in the elderly and institutionalized populations, and will increase as the population of America continues to age.

This *Clinical Practice Guideline Update* addresses major evaluative, diagnostic, treatment, and management issues of UI. It was developed under the sponsorship of the Agency for Health Care Policy and Research (AHCPR), Public Health Service, U.S. Department of Health and Human Services. To develop the guideline, AHCPR convened a multidisciplinary, expert panel of physicians, nurses, other allied health care providers, and consumers. The panel first undertook an extensive and interdisciplinary clinical review of current needs, therapeutic practices and principles, and emerging technologies for diagnosis and treatment of UI. Second, the panel conducted a comprehensive review of the field to define the existing knowledge base and critically evaluate the assumptions and common wisdom in the field. Third, the panel initiated peer review of guideline drafts with intended users in clinical sites. Comments from these reviews were assessed and used in developing the guideline.

This is an update of the *Clinical Practice Guideline on Urinary Incontinence in Adults*, first published in March 1992. This update reflects new research findings and experience with emerging technologies for UI diagnosis and treatment, and provides *specific* recommendations for diagnosing and managing adult patients with UI.

Urinary Incontinence in Adults Guideline Update Panel

Executive Summary

Urinary incontinence (UI) plagues 10–35 percent of adults and at least half of the 1.5 million nursing home residents in the United States. Because of the social stigma of UI, many sufferers do not even report the problem to a health care provider. In addition, when it is reported, many physicians and nurses, who need to be educated in this area, fail to pursue investigation of UI. As a result, this medical problem is vastly underdiagnosed and underreported.

The prevalence of UI, its toll on physical and psychological health, large variations in UI care practices and costs, and the urgent need to educate health care providers and the public about this condition prompted the selection of UI as a clinical guideline topic.

The purpose of this guideline is to improve reporting, diagnosis, and treatment of UI; reduce variations in clinical practice; educate health care providers and consumers about this condition; and, finally, encourage further biomedical, clinical, and cost research on UI. The guideline should help clinicians, caregivers, patients, and patients' families understand the assessment, management, and treatment of UI in adults. Specific reimbursement issues are not addressed.

The guideline recommendations apply to the diagnosis and treatment of acquired incontinence in ambulatory and nonambulatory patients in outpatient, inpatient, and long-term care settings. Not addressed are extraurethral UI, which is involuntary loss of urine through channels other than the urethra, UI in children, and UI due to neuropathic conditions.

To develop and update the guideline, AHCPR convened a multidisciplinary, private-sector panel of physicians, nurses, allied health professionals, and health care consumers. The panel conducted extensive literature reviews of UI in adults, heard public testimony at national hearings, and examined information gathered from consultants. It studied the effectiveness and appropriateness of diagnostic and treatment procedures for UI, how they affect outcomes important to patients, their benefits and adverse consequences, and costs incurred from their use.

The panel found evidence in the literature that the treatment of UI can improve or "cure" most patients. It determined that UI in the adult requires a comprehensive approach by health professionals in the initial evaluation and treatment with behavioral and pharmacologic interventions and requires specialists for further diagnostic evaluation and surgical intervention.

The guideline provides practice recommendations in three areas:

- **Prevention, identification, and evaluation**

  Specific risk factors for incontinence can be both identified and remediated with targeted interventions and prevention programs. The identification and documentation of UI can be improved with more thorough medical history taking, physical examination, and recordkeeping. Routine tests of lower urinary tract function should be performed for initial identification of UI. Situations that require further evaluation by qualified specialists include uncertain diagnosis, lack of correlation between symptoms and clinical findings, failure to respond to adequate therapeutic trial, hematuria without infection, presence of other comorbid conditions, and confirmation of diagnosis of incontinent patients being considered for surgical therapy. The specialized tests recommended for further diagnosis are detailed.

- ## Selection of appropriate therapy

  The guideline provides an informed framework for selecting appropriate behavioral, pharmacologic, and surgical treatments and supportive devices that can be used to manage UI. The panel concluded that behavioral techniques such as bladder retraining and pelvic muscle rehabilitation are effective, low-risk interventions that can reduce incontinence significantly in varied populations. The guideline outlines what drugs can be used effectively for certain types of incontinence, including dosages and possible side effects.

  The panel recognizes the effectiveness of surgical interventions in well-selected cases. Behavioral and pharmacologic treatments may reduce the need for surgical interventions and may be considered in the initial management.

  A new chapter on long-term management of chronic intractable UI has been added to the updated chapters from the 1992 guideline. Specific recommendations on management of patients with this condition are provided.

- ## Education of health professionals and the public

  Finally, the guideline calls for continued efforts to educate health care providers about this condition so that they are sufficiently knowledgeable to diagnose and treat it. It recommends that the public be advised to report incontinence problems once they occur and be informed that incontinence is not inevitable or shameful but is a treatable or at least manageable condition.

This is an update of the guideline, *Urinary Incontinence in Adults*, first published in March 1992. This update reflects new research findings and experience with emerging technologies and innovative approaches for UI assessment and relief. The Agency for Health Care Policy and Research and the guideline development panel welcome comments and suggestions regarding the current guideline. Please address written comments to: Director, Office of the Forum for Quality and Effectiveness in Health Care, Agency for Health Care Policy and Research, 6000 Executive Boulevard, Suite 310, Rockville, MD 20852.

1 Overview

Incidence and Prevalence

UI affects approximately 13 million Americans, with the highest prevalence in the elderly in both community and institutional settings (National Kidney and Urologic Diseases Advisory Board, 1994). The high prevalence of UI and its significant adverse physical, psychological, and financial effects clearly justify more aggressive efforts to identify, evaluate, and treat UI in all settings. Growing evidence indicates that appropriate management can reduce the morbidity and cost of UI, particularly in institutionalized populations (Ouslander, Palmer, Rovner, et al., 1993).

Although the prevalence of UI increases with age, UI should not be considered a normal part of the aging process. Reported prevalence rates of UI vary considerably, depending on the population studied, the definition of UI, and how the information is obtained (Diokno, Brock, Herzog, et al., 1990). Among the population between 15 and 64 years of age, the prevalence of UI in men ranges from 1.5 to 5 percent and in women from 10 to 30 percent (Burgio, Matthews, and Engel, 1991; Harrison and Memel, 1994). Although UI is usually regarded as a condition affecting older multiparous women, it is also common in young, nulliparous women, particularly during physical activity (Bo, Maehlum, Oseid, et al., 1989; Nygaard, Thompson, Svengalis, et al., 1994).

For noninstitutionalized persons older than 60 years of age, the prevalence of UI ranges from 15 to 35 percent, with women having twice the prevalence of men. Between 25 and 30 percent of those identified as incontinent have frequent incontinence episodes, usually daily or weekly (Burgio, Matthews, and Engel, 1991; Diokno, Brock, Brown, et al., 1986).

Survey data from caregivers of the elderly show that approximately 53 percent of the homebound elderly are incontinent (Noelker, 1987). A random sampling of hospitalized elderly patients identified 11 percent as having persistent UI at admission and 23 percent at discharge (Palmer, McCormick, Langford, et al., 1992).

UI is generally recognized as one of the major causes of institutionalization of the elderly. Among the more than 1.5 million nursing facility residents, the prevalence of UI is 50 percent or greater, with the majority of nursing home residents having frequent UI (Ouslander, Kane, and Abrass, 1982; Palmer, German, and Ouslander, 1991). The annual incidence of UI in nursing home residents who are admitted continent was recently reported to be 27 percent and is higher in males; it is strongly associated with dementia, fecal incontinence, and inability to walk and transfer independently (Ouslander, Kane, and Abrass, 1982; Palmer, German, and Ouslander, 1991).

Additional information about the prevalence of UI in nursing home residents and homebound persons is provided in Chapter 4.

Quality of Life

UI imposes a significant psychosocial impact on individuals, their families, and caregivers. UI results in a loss of self-esteem and a decrease in ability to maintain an independent lifestyle. Dependence on caregivers for activities of daily life increases as incontinence worsens. Consequently, excursions outside the home, social interaction with friends and family, and sexual activity may be restricted or avoided entirely (Grimby, Milsom, Molander, et al., 1993; Harris, 1986; Noelker, 1987). Quality-of-life and symptom distress questionnaires for women with UI have been validated for use (Shumaker, Wyman, Uebersax, et al., 1994; Uebersax, Wyman, Shumaker, et al., 1995).

Underreporting/Undertreatment

Fewer than half of individuals with UI living in the community consult health care providers about the problem (Burgio, Ives, Locher, et al., 1994). The reasons for this could be the availability of absorbent products, low expectations of benefit from reporting the condition to health care providers, and lack of information regarding management options. There is a lack of understanding about UI, especially among men, those age 85 or older, and those with lower levels of education (Branch, Walker, Wetle, et al., 1994).

Studies show significant variation in performance of adequate examination, assessment, and management of UI. UI is often undetected and underreported by hospital and nursing home personnel, masking its true extent and clinical impact and reducing the opportunity for effective management. Assessment tools with cue words for continence status significantly improve identification of UI in nursing homes and increase the opportunity for effective management (Palmer, McCormick, Langford, et al., 1992).

Risk Factors and Prevention

The incidence of incontinence is sufficiently high that the development of an effective prevention program would reduce new cases of incontinence in community-dwelling women alone by approximately 50,000 cases annually (Siu, Beers, and Morgenstern, 1993). There is good evidence that specific risk factors for incontinence can be both identified and remediated with targeted interventions. However, no controlled clinical trial data exist showing that these interventions reduce incontinence incidence, severity, or prevalence. Table 1 provides a summary of risk factors associated with incontinence that have been documented in the literature. Some of the risk factors for UI are discussed further in Chapter 2. Only one reference has been listed for each risk factor, although in most cases multiple studies have described the same factor. Several of the studies described interventions that have modified these risk factors successfully.

Table 1. Risk factors associated with incontinence

Risk factor	Reference
Immobility/chronic degenerative disease	Ouslander, Palmer, Rovner, et al., 1993; Adams, Lorish, Cushing, et al., 1994
Impaired cognition	Morris, Browne, and Saltmarche, 1992; Skelly and Flint, 1995
Medications	Dwyer and Teele, 1992
Morbid obesity	Bump and McClish, 1994
Diuretics	Diokno, Brock, Herzog, et al., 1990
Smoking	Bump and McClish, 1994
Fecal impaction	Resnick and Yalla, 1985
Delirium	Resnick, 1988
Low fluid intake	Colling, Owen, and McCreedy, 1994
Environmental barriers	Wyman, Elswick, Ory, et al., 1993
High-impact physical activities	Nygaard, Thompson, Svengalis, et al., 1994
Diabetes	Appell and Baum, 1990
Stroke	Benbow, Sangster, and Barer, 1991
Estrogen depletion	Burns, Nochajski, and Pranifoff, 1993
Pelvic muscle weakness	Burns, Nochajski, and Pranifoff, 1993
Childhood nocturnal enuresis	Moore, Richmond, and Parys, 1991
Race	Burgio, Matthews, and Engel, 1991
Pregnancy/vaginal delivery/ episiotomy	Foldspang, Mommsen, Lam, et al., 1992; Klein, Gauthier, Robbins, et al., 1994

Costs

A recent estimate of the direct costs of caring for persons of all ages with incontinence is $11.2 billion annually in the community and $5.2 billion in nursing homes (based on 1994 dollars) (Hu, 1994). This cost estimate is more than 60 percent greater than a previous estimate (Hu, 1990), an increase greater than that for the cost of services in the medical care sector. Data show that costs of providing care for UI vary widely (Baker and Bice, 1995; Hu, Gabelko, Weiss, et al., 1994).

The guideline does not address specific reimbursement issues, which are being evaluated by other groups (National Kidney and Urologic Diseases Advisory Board, 1994).

Purpose and Scope

The original *Clinical Practice Guideline on Urinary Incontinence in Adults* was published in March 1992. The purpose and scope of the 1992 guideline and the methodology for its development are outlined below. The process used for updating the original guideline, which resulted in the publication of this *Clinical Practice Guideline Update on Urinary Incontinence in Adults: Acute and Chronic Management*, is also outlined.

1992 Guideline

The original UI guideline panel defined UI as involuntary loss of urine that is sufficient to be a problem. The panel agreed that the guideline, which sought to improve the care of incontinent adults, should be directed toward acquired incontinence in ambulatory and nonambulatory patients in outpatient, inpatient, home care, and long-term care settings. Extraurethral UI, which is involuntary loss of urine through channels other than the urethra, was not addressed in the document. The guideline was targeted to all practitioners who encounter UI, with the primary outcome of elimination or reduction of UI.

The original panel also agreed on the components of the evaluation and management of UI, which were considered to be the management model for the guideline. The original guideline made seven broad-based recommendations, as follows:

1. Improve the education and dissemination of UI diagnosis and treatment alternatives to the public and to health care providers.

2. Educate the consumer to report incontinence problems once they occur.

3. Improve the detection and documentation of UI through better medical histories and health care recordkeeping.

4. Establish appropriate basic evaluation and criteria for further evaluation.

5. Delineate the steps of appropriate management.

6. Where appropriate, reduce variations among health care providers, while maintaining flexibility to individualize treatment to individual patients.

7. Encourage further biomedical and clinical research on prevention, diagnosis, and treatment of UI in adults and encourage further research into the costs of UI diagnosis and treatment and the cost benefit of prevention programs.

The original panel conducted an extensive literature review on UI in adults, heard public testimony at a national hearing, and reviewed information from consultants. It also sought further evidence of the costs of UI, variations in practice and payments, the prevalence of incontinence in hospitals, and the incidence of UI in outpatient, rehabilitation, and home settings.

Previous research data and expert opinions helped to provide insight into the problem within communities, acute care facilities, and nursing homes. The draft guideline was also extensively peer-reviewed by individual experts and representatives of the various professional and public organizations, and many of their recommendations were incorporated into the document.

The panel found evidence that treatment of UI is effective in most people; however, the condition was underreported, services were improperly or poorly documented, and major variations in diagnosis and treatment were identified as significant problems.

The original UI panel also recommended that review of the guideline respond to new developments in UI research, training, product developments, practice, and patient participation. Because of the magnitude of literature produced each year, the panel recommended that the guideline be updated annually.

Updating the Guideline

Because the recommendations were so broad-based, AHCPR recommended updating the guideline to include recent literature and to provide specific recommendations for managing UI in adults. AHCPR provided the general parameters for this update of the guideline. An update can be in the form of amendments to the guideline or a more complete update and reprinting. In the months following release of a guideline, the Office of the Forum surveys subsequently published scientific literature in the topic areas addressed by the guideline to determine the volume of new scientific evidence, its quality, and the likelihood that such information would cause a change in the guideline recommendations. Comments are also solicited from the public regarding the availability of new scientific evidence or new technologies that may warrant an update. Other relevant information may be obtained from evaluation studies conducted to examine the implementation or effects of the guidelines. When sufficient data are obtained to indicate that a guideline update may be needed, a public meeting to address the need for and timing of an update is convened.

After reviewing and analyzing the findings from the update literature review and analysis since 1992, the Office of the Forum recommended a complete update and reprinting of the guideline. The primary goals of the update process were to present new developments in UI research that affect diagnosis and management of the condition and to develop specific recommendations for each assessment and treatment method. The algorithm for management of UI in primary care was revised to reflect the findings and recommendations of the panel (see Attachment A).

Methodology for Updating the Guideline

The following specific activities were undertaken to update the original UI guideline.

Formation of the Panel

AHCPR initiated formation of the update panel and appointed its chairperson and members. A notice published in the *Federal Register* invited nominations of new candidates to replace the departing panel members. The original panel chairs reviewed nominations received by AHCPR and provided their recommendations to AHCPR to replace departing members. Following these recommendations, AHCPR selected and appointed the replacement members for the update period. The update panel comprised 16 members representing the multidisciplinary areas included in the original panel—the departing cochairs were replaced by two of the original panel members, six other original members remained, and eight new members joined. Several consultants with expertise in nursing and primary care, methodology, literature review and analysis, and cost analysis, as well as a representative of the Centers for Disease Control and Prevention (CDC), were appointed to the panel. Over the course of the update process the panel also sought the advice and assistance of 22 technical specialists to evaluate the literature and develop revisions to the original guideline.

Public Comment and Peer Review

An open forum was held September 20, 1993, to give interested individuals, organizations, and agencies the opportunity to present written or verbal testimony. Later in the process, drafts of the revised guideline were sent out for peer review. AHCPR selected peer reviewers from those who had expressed interest in the guideline, participated in the open forum, or were nominated by professional organizations or panel members. The 22 technical specialists were included among the peer reviewers. The reviewers were asked to evaluate the comprehensiveness of the literature review as well as the panel's findings and recommendations. The panel incorporated their comments into the final revision of the guideline.

Literature Search

The panel initiated a comprehensive literature search of topics relating to adult UI. The bibliography from the original guideline was the starting point for this literature search.

The search for literature published since the final literature search conducted for the 1992 guideline was performed through the National Library of Medicine. Over the course of the update process, three searches were conducted. Abstracts of approximately 1,500 articles that met the search criteria were each independently evaluated by panel members for scientific quality and relevance to the guideline update. Approximately 1,200 articles were obtained for further evaluation.

Additional articles came from panel members, from the open forum process, and from unsolicited sources. All articles were entered into a comprehensive bibliography, classified by topic, and screened systematically to determine if they contained information of use to the update panel.

Literature Review and Data Abstraction

The articles were categorized and assigned to corresponding subcommittees for screening and further review. These categories were prevalence, prevention, and quality of life; cost; causes and diagnostic evaluation; behavioral treatment; pharmacological treatment; surgery; supportive devices; and professional and public education. The methodology to identify and evaluate the scientific evidence on each assessment and treatment method included a systematic evaluation of each study's quality and its applicability to adult patients with UI. The panel screened all articles, using minimum article selection criteria to select articles for data abstraction. The panel subcommittees used a common data abstraction method, but because of the varied nature of the subject, each subcommittee determined its own inclusion/exclusion criteria. The pharmacology subcommittee restricted review to clinical efficacy studies of drugs likely to be available in the United States. Because few such studies exist in other areas, it was not possible to place similar restrictions on the review of behavioral and surgical interventions. Minimum criteria generally required that articles represent a designed study (not a case report) with outcome defined in some manner. The articles selected were then sent to technical specialists for review for data abstraction and for confirmation of the data abstraction process. The technical specialists followed the same data abstraction process to evaluate the quality and to abstract pertinent data from each article. The articles on behavioral, pharmacologic, and surgical treatments were further reviewed and summaries of results (with total number of subjects and a range or average of improvement or success rates) provided. The papers on diagnostic, supportive, and health education were not judged applicable for meta-analysis. The panel then reviewed the available data to decide how much weight to give each study in developing the recommendation statements for the update guideline.

Outcome Measures

The panel was aware of the limits of and issues surrounding current outcome measures while evaluating the available data on assessment and treatment methods for UI. The current outcome measure of UI treatment is to stop urine leakage or to reduce its amount, frequency, or both. Measuring urine leakage or wetting is difficult, however. The panel agreed that UI outcome can be measured in many domains (e.g., patients' opinions, diaries, pad tests, quality-of-life scales, urodynamic tests) and that each of these domains is continuous and not discrete. The International Continence Society and other groups are considering standardization of outcome measures.

The wide variability in outcomes measured in different articles made it difficult to choose a single outcome measure to assess treatment. Because the subjective outcome of "cure," improvement, or both was cited in studies much more often than objective measures, this was the outcome the panel generally relied on. When sufficient articles presented results on incontinent episodes, these were also noted.

Developing the Guideline Recommendations

To develop recommendations for each assessment and treatment method, the panel considered (1) the quality and amount of evidence, (2) the consistency of findings among studies, (3) the clinical applicability of the evidence to adult patients with UI, and (4) the evidence on harms or costs.

Specific recommendation statements were developed by the panel collectively. The panel rated the strength of evidence supporting each recommendation, based on the following criteria:

A   The recommendation is supported by scientific evidence from properly designed and implemented controlled trials providing statistical results that consistently support the guideline statement.

B   The recommendation is supported by scientific evidence from properly designed and implemented clinical series that support the guideline statement.

C   The recommendation is supported by expert opinion.

Please note that these ratings represent the strength of the supporting research evidence, not the strength of the recommendation itself. The strength of each recommendation is conveyed in the language describing it.

Clinical Algorithm

The overview algorithm in Attachment A provides the health care provider with a visual display of the conceptual organization, procedural flow, decision points, and preferred management pathways discussed in the guideline.

2 Identifying and Evaluating Urinary Incontinence

Symptoms and Subtypes

UI can be caused by anatomic, physiologic, and pathologic (genitourinary) factors affecting the urinary tract, as well as external (nongenitourinary) factors. Multiple and interacting factors often contribute to UI development, especially in frail, older patients (Ouslander and Bruskewitz, 1989). In such patients, the diagnostic evaluation must be comprehensive, focusing not only on the lower urinary tract but also on the patient's general medical and functional status.

Several conditions that cause or contribute to UI are potentially reversible (see Table 2). Management of one or more of these conditions can sometimes lead to the resolution of the UI. This potentially reversible type of UI has been referred to as transient incontinence. In other patients, treatment of these conditions will reduce the severity of UI but will not totally resolve it. Several different nosologies have been used to classify the various types of UI. The classification of subtypes of UI used here is based on symptoms so as to facilitate use of this guideline by primary health care providers. Often, classifications used by specialists incorporate primarily pathophysiologic characteristics.

Urge Incontinence

The symptom of urge incontinence is the involuntary loss of urine associated with a strong desire to void (urgency). Urge incontinence is usually, but not always, associated with the urodynamic finding of involuntary detrusor contractions, referred to as detrusor instability (DI). Although DI can be associated with neurologic disorders, it also occurs in individuals who appear to be neurologically normal. The uninhibited bladder contractions associated with DI can cause UI with and without symptoms of urgency; it can also cause symptoms of urgency without concomitant incontinence (Fantl, Wyman, McClish, et al., 1991). When a causative neurologic lesion is established, the DI is called detrusor hyperreflexia (DH) (Abrams, Blaivas, Stanton, et al., 1988). A common neurologic disorder associated with DH is stroke. In patients with suprasacral spinal cord lesions and multiple sclerosis, DH is commonly accompanied by detrusor sphincter dyssynergia (DSD) (inappropriate contraction of the external sphincter with detrusor contraction). This can result in the development of urinary retention, vesicoureteral reflux, and subsequent renal damage (McGuire, Woodside, Borden, et al., 1981).

Another urodynamic diagnosis associated with the symptom of urge incontinence in frail, elderly patients is detrusor hyperactivity with impaired bladder contractility (DHIC) (Resnick and Yalla, 1985). Patients with DHIC

Table 2. Identification and management of reversible conditions that cause or contribute to urinary incontinence

Condition	Management
Conditions affecting the lower urinary tract	
Urinary tract infection (symptomatic with frequency, urgency, dysuria, etc.)	Antimicrobial therapy
Atrophic vaginitis/urethritis	Oral or topical estrogen (see Chapter 3 section on Pharmacologic Treatment)
Pregnancy/vaginal delivery/episiotomy	Behavioral intervention. Avoid surgical therapy postpartum as condition may be self-limiting
Postprostatectomy	Behavioral intervention. Avoid surgical therapy until clear condition will not resolve
Stool impaction	Disimpaction; appropriate use of stool softeners, bulk-forming agents, and laxatives if necessary; implement high fiber intake, adequate mobility and fluid intake
Drug side effects[a]	
Diuretics: causing polyuria, frequency, and urgency	With all medications discontinue or change therapy, as clinically possible. Dosage reduction or modification (e.g., flexible scheduling of rapid-acting diuretics) may also help
Caffeine: causing aggravation or precipitation of UI	
Anticholinergic agents: causing urinary retention, overflow incontinence, impaction	

Psychotropics
   Antidepressants: causing anticholinergic actions, sedation
   Antipsychotics: causing anticholinergic actions, sedation, rigidity, and immobility
   Sedatives/hypnotics/CNS depressants: causing sedation, delirium, immobility, muscle relaxation	

Narcotic analgesics: causing urinary retention, fecal impaction, sedation, delirium	
Alpha-adrenergic blockers: causing urethral relaxation	

Table 2. (continued)

Condition	Management
Alpha-adrenergic agonists: causing urinary retention (present in many cold and diet over-the-counter (OTC) preparations)	
Beta-adrenergic agonists: causing urinary retention	
Calcium channel blockers: causing urinary retention	
Alcohol: causing polyuria, frequency, urgency, sedation, delirium, immobility	
Increased urine production	
Metabolic (hyperglycemia, hypercalcemia)	Better control of diabetes mellitus. Therapy for hypercalcemia depends on underlying cause.
Excess fluid intake	Reduction in intake of diuretic fluids (e.g., caffeinated beverages)
Volume overload Venous insufficiency with edema	Support stocking Leg elevation Sodium restriction Diuretic therapy
Congestive heart failure	Medical therapy
Impaired ability or willingness to reach a toilet	
Delirium	Diagnosis and treatment of underlying cause(s) of acute confusional state
Chronic illness, injury, or restraint that interferes with mobility	Regular toileting Use of toilet substitutes Environmental alterations (e.g., bedside commode, urinal)
Psychological	Remove restraints if possible. Appropriate pharmacologic and/or nonpharmacologic treatment

[a]Many side effects are seen with over-the-counter (OTC) drugs, the use of which may not be reported by some patients.

have involuntary detrusor contractions, yet must strain to empty their bladders either incompletely or completely. Clinically, patients with DHIC generally have symptoms of urge incontinence and an elevated postvoid residual (PVR) volume, but they may also have symptoms of obstruction, stress incontinence, or overflow incontinence. DHIC must be distinguished from other types of UI because it can mimic them, resulting in inappropriate diagnosis and treatment.

Stress Incontinence

The symptom of stress urinary incontinence (SUI) presents clinically as the involuntary loss of urine during coughing, sneezing, laughing, or other physical activities that increase intra-abdominal pressure. SUI is defined as urine loss coincident with an increase in intra-abdominal pressure, in the absence of a detrusor contraction or an overdistended bladder. The most common cause of SUI in women is urethral hypermobility, or significant displacement of the urethra and bladder neck during exertion when intra-abdominal pressure is raised.

SUI may also be caused by an intrinsic urethral sphincter deficiency (ISD), which may be due to congenital sphincter weakness in patients with myelomeningocele, epispadias, or pelvic denervation, or may be acquired after prostatectomy, trauma, radiation therapy, or a sacral cord lesion. In women, ISD is commonly associated with multiple incontinence surgical procedures, as well as with hypoestrogenism, aging, or both. In this condition, the urethral sphincter is unable to generate enough resistance to retain urine in the bladder, especially during stress maneuvers (Blaivas, 1985; Staskin, Zimmern, Hadley, et al., 1985). Patients with ISD often leak continuously or with minimal exertion. In some patients, stress incontinence results from coexisting ISD and hypermobility of the urethra and bladder neck.

Mixed Incontinence

It is not unusual for patients to present with a combination of urge and stress incontinence (Fantl, Wyman, McClish, et al., 1990; Ouslander, Hepps, Raz, et al., 1986). When both symptoms are present, the incontinence is called mixed UI. Mixed UI is common in women, especially older women. Often, however, one symptom (urge or stress) is more bothersome to the patient than the other. Identifying the most bothersome symptom is important in targeting diagnostic and therapeutic interventions.

Overflow Incontinence

Involuntary loss of urine associated with overdistension of the bladder is termed overflow incontinence. This type of incontinence may have a variety of presentations, including frequent or constant dribbling, or urge or stress incontinence symptoms. Overflow UI may be caused by an underactive or acontractile detrusor, or to bladder outlet or urethral obstruction leading to overdistension and overflow. The bladder may be underactive or acontractile secondary to drugs, neurologic conditions such as diabetic neuropathy, low spinal cord injury, or radical pelvic surgery that interrupts the motor innervation of the detrusor muscle. The detrusor muscle may also be underactive from idiopathic causes.

In men, overflow incontinence associated with obstruction is commonly caused by prostatic hyperplasia and, less frequently, prostatic carcinoma or urethral stricture. Although an outlet obstruction is rare in women, it can occur as a complication of an anti-incontinence operation and because of severe pelvic organ prolapse, in which the organ involved protrudes to or beyond the vaginal orifice (e.g., prolapsing cystocele, uterine prolapse). In patients with suprasacral spinal cord injury or multiple sclerosis, DSD can cause obstruction when the external sphincter muscle inappropriately and involuntarily contracts rather than relaxes at the same time the detrusor contracts (Blaivas, 1985).

Other Causes and Types

Functional Incontinence. Urine loss may be caused by factors outside the lower urinary tract such as chronic impairment of physical or cognitive functioning, or both, a condition commonly termed "functional incontinence" (Williams and Pannill, 1982). This diagnosis should be one of exclusion, however, because some immobile and cognitively impaired individuals have other types and causes of UI that may respond to specific therapies (Skelly and Flint, 1995). For example, most nursing home residents have not only functional limitations that interfere with their ability to toilet but also urge UI with detrusor instability or DH. In addition, UI can often be improved or "cured" by improving the patient's functional status, treating other medical conditions, discontinuing certain types of medication, adjusting the hydration status, reducing environmental barriers, or all of the above—even if a lower urinary tract abnormality is present.

Unconscious or Reflex Incontinence. Urine loss may also occur without any warning or sensory awareness such as in paraplegics and some patients without overt neurologic dysfunction. This condition, which also has been termed unconscious incontinence, presents as either postmicturitional or constant (continuous) dribbling. Extraurethral UI (i.e., fistulas), UI in children, and neuropathic conditions are not specifically addressed in this guideline.

Another urodynamic finding that may be associated with UI is decreased bladder compliance. This abnormal bladder condition may result from radiation cystitis, inflammatory bladder conditions such as chemical cystitis or interstitial cystitis, and some neurologic bladder disorders such as those that occur following radical pelvic surgery and in myelomeningocele. Many of the patients with a nonneurogenic etiology for their decreased bladder compliance (e.g., chemical or radiation cystitis) have severe urgency associated with bladder hypersensitivity and with no demonstrable DI. This is termed "sensory urgency." Both loss of bladder wall elasticity and lack of bladder accommodation produce a steep rise in intravesical pressure during bladder filling without detrusor contraction. In patients in whom the urethral sphincter mechanism may already be compromised by the condition that produced the inelastic bladder (e.g., radiation, neurologic dysfunction), the abnormal increase in bladder pressure may overcome the urethral pressure and produce UI. A major concern in patients with a poorly compliant bladder, especially those who are neurologically impaired, is the development of vesicoureteral reflux and hydronephrosis.

Identifying Urinary Incontinence

Because many people with UI delay or do not seek professional help (Herzog, Fultz, Normolle, et al., 1989; Norton, MacDonald, Sedgwick, et al., 1988), primary health care providers should question their patients regularly to identify UI. Open-ended requests such as "Tell me about the problems you are having with your bladder" and "Tell me about the trouble you are having holding your urine (water)" are a useful initial approach. If the patient responds negatively, more specific questions such as "How often do you lose urine when you don't want to?" and "How often do you wear a pad or other protective device to collect your urine?" may help identify UI. In licensed nursing facilities, assessment of continence status using the Minimum Data Set (MDS) is required within 14 days of admission and every 3 months thereafter (Morris, Hawes, Murphy, et al., 1990).

If UI is identified by questioning, detecting an odor, observing wetness, or by a patient complaint, and represents a problem for the patient or caregiver, evaluation should be undertaken as described below.

General Principles of Diagnostic Evaluation

Health care providers are encouraged to be knowledgeable about and initiate the basic evaluation of patients with UI. (Strength of Evidence = C.)

When UI is a problem for the patient or caregiver, the patient should undergo a basic evaluation by a health care provider. UI has traditionally been evaluated by specialists, including gynecologists and urologists, and in some rehabilitation settings, by physiatrists. Given the high prevalence of UI in the general population, however, limiting UI evaluation and management to these specialists is not feasible. The panel encourages primary health care providers, such as family physicians, general internists, geriatricians, nurse practitioners and specialists, and physician assistants, to be knowledgeable about and able to initiate the basic evaluation of UI.

Basic Evaluation

All patients with UI should undergo a basic evaluation that includes a history, physical examination, measurement of postvoid residual volume, and urinalysis. (Strength of Evidence = B.)

Risk factors that are associated with UI should be identified and attempts made to modify them. (Strength of Evidence = B.)

Purpose

UI is a symptom and not a condition in itself. Thus, the purposes of the basic evaluation are to

1. Confirm the presence of UI.

2. Identify conditions, including potentially reversible ones (see Table 2), that may be contributing to the UI.

3. Identify patients who require further evaluation before any therapeutic interventions are attempted and patients who may receive initial treatment without further testing.

4. Identify a presumptive diagnosis, if possible.

Components

The basic evaluation should include a history, physical examination, estimation of PVR volume, and urinalysis. The basic evaluation may not be appropriate for every patient, and every health care provider may not have the background to complete this assessment for some patients. At any time during the basic evaluation, the health care provider may refer the patient for further evaluation by a specialist.

History. The history should include (1) a focused medical, neurologic, and genitourinary history that includes an assessment of risk factors (see Table 1) and a review of medications (including nonprescription medications) and (2) a detailed exploration of the symptoms of the UI and associated symptoms and factors, including

- Duration and characteristics of UI (stress, urge, dribbling, others).

- Most bothersome symptom(s) to the patient (which may be especially important in guiding therapy and determining response).

- Frequency, timing, and amount of continent voids and incontinent episodes.

- Precipitants of incontinence (e.g., situational antecedents, cough, certain types of exercises, surgery, injury, previous pelvic radiation therapy, trauma, new onset of diseases, new medications).

- Other lower urinary tract symptoms (e.g., nocturia, dysuria, hesitancy, poor or interrupted stream, straining, hematuria, suprapubic or perineal pain).

- Fluid intake pattern, including caffeine-containing or other diuretic fluids.

- Alterations in bowel habits or sexual function.

- Previous treatments and their effects on UI.

- Amount and types of pads, briefs, and protective devices.

- Expectations for outcomes of treatment.

- A bladder record.

- A mental status evaluation and assessment of mobility, living environment, and social factors, especially in elderly patients.

Bladder records are helpful supplements to the history in many patients (Diokno, Wells, and Brink, 1987; Larson and Victor, 1992; Wyman, Choi, Harkins, et al., 1988). These written records are used to determine the frequency, timing, and amount of voiding, as well as other factors associated with UI. Such a record can be kept by the patient or a caregiver for a few days before the basic evaluation. The record may provide clues about the underlying cause of UI, as well as information on fluid intake and voiding patterns that may be helpful for behavioral interventions, and can serve as a baseline to gauge severity and treatment efficacy (see sample records, Attachments B and C).

A mental status examination should be performed when appropriate. Assessment of mobility and living environment is also especially important in certain individuals. Questions should be asked about access to toilets or toilet substitutes, and about social factors such as living arrangements, social contacts, or caregiver involvement (Williams and Gaylord, 1990).

Physical Examination. The physical examination should include the following:

- *General examination* if indicated to detect conditions such as edema that may contribute to nocturia and nocturnal UI; to detect neurologic abnormalities that may suggest multiple sclerosis, stroke, spinal cord compression, or other neurologic conditions; and to assess mobility, cognition, and manual dexterity related to toileting skills among frail and functionally impaired patients (Williams and Gaylord, 1990).

- *Abdominal examination* to check for diastasis rectii, organomegaly, masses, peritonitis, fluid collections, and so on. Abnormality of abdominal contents may influence intra-abdominal pressure and detrusor physiology.

- *Rectal examination* to test for perineal sensation, sphincter tone (both resting and active), fecal impaction, or rectal mass, and to evaluate the consistency and contour of the prostate in men. The size of the prostate on digital examination does not exclude or imply obstruction and is usually helpful only for the surgeon in determining the surgical approach if an operation is contemplated.

- *Genital examination in men* to evaluate skin condition and detect abnormalities of the foreskin, glans penis, and perineal skin.

- *Pelvic examination in women* to assess perineal skin condition, genital atrophy, pelvic organ prolapse (cystocele, rectocele, uterine prolapse), pelvic mass, paravaginal muscle tone, or other abnormalities. Palpation of the anterior vaginal wall and urethra may elicit urethral discharge or tenderness that suggests a urethral diverticulum, carcinoma, or inflammatory condition of the urethra. Pelvic organ prolapse may not relate to urinary symptoms, especially in the elderly (Ouslander, Hepps, Raz, et al., 1986).

- *Direct observation of urine loss* using the cough stress test. Observation of urine loss can be performed by having the individual cough vigorously while the examiner observes for urine loss from the urethra. Optimally, testing should be done when the patient's bladder is full but before the patient has a precipitant urge to void (Kadar, 1988). In women who are being evaluated for specific treatments for stress incontinence, this test is important for objective demonstration of urine loss and identification of provoking factors. In other patients, particularly those with physical or cognitive impairment, direct observation may be difficult to carry out, and this documentation may not be critical in determining initial treatment of incontinence. If an instantaneous leakage occurs with cough, then SUI is likely; if leakage is delayed or persists after the cough, DI should be suspected. If the test is initially performed in the lithotomy position and no leakage is observed, the test should be repeated in the upright position (Kadar, 1988). If bladder filling is needed to perform stress testing, it may be conveniently performed in conjunction with the catheterization method of measurement of PVR volume.

Estimation of PVR Volume. Accurate measurement of PVR can be accomplished either by catheterization or by pelvic ultrasound (Coombes and Millard, 1994; Haylen, Frazer, and MacDonald, 1989; Ireton, Krieger, Cardenas, et al., 1990). Some health care providers may use abdominal palpation or bimanual pelvic examination to suspect elevated PVR; however, the exact amount of volume or confirmation usually requires other methods (catheterization, ultrasound) (Norton, Peattie, and Stanton, 1989).

Before PVR is measured, the patient should void in the most comfortable and private environment possible. Voiding can be observed at this time to detect signs of hesitancy, straining, or slow or interrupted stream, which may indicate urethral obstruction, a bladder contractility problem, or both.

Measurement of PVR volume is generally done within a few minutes after voiding by catheterizing the patient or by pelvic ultrasound. Review of the literature failed to indicate a specific maximum PVR volume considered normal, nor is there any documentation of the minimal PVR considered abnormal. In general, PVRs of less than 50 mL are considered adequate bladder emptying. Repetitive PVRs ranging from 100 to 200 or higher are considered inadequate emptying. Clinical judgment must be exercised and all other clinical information included in interpreting the significance of PVR volume, especially in the intermediate range of 50–199 mL.

The PVR urine may be influenced by such factors as the volume voided before PVR measurement, whether the patient is "ready" to void or strains to void, the efforts made to drain the bladder completely, and the environment or clinical setting. Because PVR volume may vary, one measurement of PVR may not be sufficient and repeated measurements may be of value in some patients.

Urethral catheterization in men with prostate obstruction may cause urinary tract infection. Therefore, catheterization in men should be performed only with clear indication and by a health care provider who is prepared to manage abnormal findings.

An alternative to catheterization is the use of pelvic ultrasound. Portable ultrasound devices that estimate PVR with reasonable accuracy are now available (Ireton, Krieger, Cardenas, et al., 1990; Ouslander, Simmons, Tuico, et al., 1994; Topper, Holliday, and Fernie, 1993).

Urinalysis. This test is used to detect conditions that are associated with or contributing to UI such as hematuria (suggestive of infection, cancer, or stone), glucosuria (which may cause polyuria and contribute to UI symptoms), pyuria, and bacteriuria, as well as glycosuria and proteinuria. If catheterization is performed for PVR measurement, a sample of the residual urine can be used for the urinalysis and microscopic examination. Careful cleaning of the glans penis in men and the periurethral area in women with an antiseptic solution allows collection of a spontaneously voided specimen that accurately reflects bladder urine.

Dipstick methods are available to detect bacteriuria and pyuria. The diagnostic accuracy of these methods varies considerably among methods and different patient populations (Lachs, Nachamkin, Edelstein, et al., 1992). Therefore, urine cultures should be obtained in incontinent patients when dipstick tests indicate infection or when symptoms suggest infection.

Among chronically incontinent nursing home residents, eradication of bacteriuria (with or without pyuria) has no effect on morbidity, mortality, or the severity of UI (Boscia, Kobasa, Abrutyn, et al., 1986). Thus, unless UI is of recent onset, has recently worsened, or is accompanied by other symptoms of infection (e.g., dysuria, hematuria, fever, sudden decline in mental or physical functioning), bacteriuria (with or without pyuria) does not need to be treated in this patient population. Among noninstitutionalized patients, the relationship of bacteriuria (with or without pyuria) to UI is unclear. Further research is needed to clarify this relationship. Until such data are available, infection should be treated when the incontinent patient is initially evaluated and the effect observed before further diagnostic or therapeutic interventions are undertaken (Ouslander, 1989).

Supplementary Assessments. The use of blood tests (BUN, creatinine, glucose, and calcium) and urine cytology in the assessment of the incontinent patient was also evaluated.

Blood testing (BUN, creatinine, glucose, and calcium) is recommended if compromised renal function is suspected or if polyuria (in the absence of diuretics) is present. (Strength of Evidence = C.)

Blood tests that may be helpful in the basic evaluation of the incontinent patient include creatinine levels in patients suspected of having obstruction, noncompliant bladders, or urinary retention. However, normal creatinine levels do not rule out hydronephrosis. Patients with polyuria in the absence of diuretic agents should be evaluated for excess intake (diabetes insipidus), hyperglycemia, and hypercalcemia if indicated.

Urine cytology is not recommended in the routine evaluation of the incontinent patient. (Strength of Evidence = B.)

There is no evidence in the literature to support urine cytology testing in patients with UI. Individuals with incontinence are at no higher risk of bladder cancer than the continent population (Mohr, Offord, Owen, et al., 1986). Urine cytology is a poor screening test for bladder cancer, with sensitivities ranging from approximately 20–70 percent (Curling, Broome, and Gendry, 1986; Murphy, 1990; Rife, Farrow, and Utz, 1979). Patients with hematuria (2–5 RBC/hpf) or acute onset of irritative voiding symptoms in the absence of urinary tract infection (UTI) require cystoscopy and cytology to exclude bladder neoplasm (Utz and Zincke, 1974).

Further Evaluation

After the basic evaluation, treatment for the presumed type of urinary incontinence should be initiated unless there is an indication for further evaluation. (Strength of Evidence = B.)

After the basic evaluation, all incontinent patients in whom transient (reversible) causes of UI have been detected should be treated appropriately (see Table 2). If UI persists after the transient causes are identified and treated, further evaluation may be helpful before therapy is initiated.

Examples of patients who may not need further evaluation before initiating treatment follow:

- Patients with SUI, normal PVR volume, and no complicating features.

- Patients with urge UI, normal PVR volume, and no complicating features.

- Women with mixed urge–stress UI with normal PVR volume and no complicating features for whom behavioral or pharmacologic therapy, or both, is preferred.

Initial management options for these patients are outlined in Table 3. Patients requiring further evaluation include those who meet any of the criteria in Table 4. Because of their general medical condition, some of these patients may not be appropriate for further evaluation, particularly if it is not desired by the patient or feasible.

After the basic evaluation and initial treatment, patients who fail or those who are not appropriate for treatment based on presumptive diagnosis should undergo further evaluation. (Strength of Evidence = C.)

The objectives of further evaluation are as follows:

- Identify the specific cause or causes of UI with reproduction of leakage during testing.

- Identify conditions that cause similar symptoms but require different treatments, such as outlet obstruction, detrusor muscle weakness, urethral hypermobility, ISD, and urethral diverticulum.

- Detect functional, neurologic, or anatomic lesions affecting the lower urinary tract.

- Help obtain specific information necessary for choosing the appropriate therapy.

- Identify risk factors that may influence the outcome of a specific treatment.

Specialized Tests

Specialized tests are not intended to be part of the basic evaluation of UI. (Strength of Evidence = B.)

Numerous specialized diagnostic tests are available, and the evaluation must be tailored to the question to be answered. Specialized tests include the following:

- Urodynamic tests.

- Endoscopic tests.

- Imaging tests.

Table 5 summarizes the major symptoms of incontinence, associated factors, conditions, and diagnostic test options. Although the primary care physician is not expected to be an expert in these techniques, health care providers should be familiar with the diagnostic tests that may be used in evaluating the symptoms of UI.

Table 3. Management options after basic evaluation

Type of UI	Characteristics	Management options

Urge	Detrusor instability
	With normal PVR, no complicating factors
		Behavioral techniques
		  Bladder training
		  Pelvic muscle rehabilitation
		  Other (e.g., fluid management)
		
		Pharmacologic interventions
		  Anticholinergic medications, tricyclic antidepressants as alternative

Stress	With normal PVR, no complicating factors	Behavioral techniques
		  Pelvic muscle rehabilitation
		  Bladder training
		
		Pharmacologic techniques
		  Alpha-adrenergic medications or tricyclic antidepressants; estrogen; combination if needed
		
		Surgical techniques
		  Uncomplicated, nonrecurrent SUI due to hypermobility

Mixed (Urge-Stress)	With normal PVR, no complicating factors	Combinations of above excluding surgical options in most cases

Table 4. Criteria for further evaluation[a]

- Uncertain diagnosis and inability to develop a reasonable treatment plan based on the basic diagnostic evaluation. Uncertainty in diagnosis may occur when there is lack of correlation between symptoms and clinical findings.

- Failure to respond to the patient's satisfaction to an adequate therapeutic trial, and the patient is interested in pursuing further therapy.

- Consideration of surgical intervention, particularly if previous surgery failed or the patient is a high surgical risk.

- Hematuria without infection.

- The presence of other comorbid conditions, such as

  - incontinence associated with recurrent symptomatic UTI
  - persistent symptoms of difficult bladder emptying
  - history of previous anti-incontinence surgery or radical pelvic surgery
  - beyond hymen and symptomatic pelvic prolapse
  - prostate nodule, asymmetry, or other suspicion of prostate cancer
  - abnormal PVR urine
  - neurologic condition, such as multiple sclerosis and spinal cord lesions or injury.

[a]Some patients who meet the criteria may not be appropriate for further evaluation and treatment if such evaluation and/or treatment is not desired by or feasible for the patient.

Table 5. Diagnostic test options[a]

Type of UI	Mechanism	Associated factors	Diagnostic test options
Urge	Unstable bladder or detrusor instability (DI)	No neurologic deficit	Simple or multichannel CMG with or without EMG
	Detrusor hyperreflexia (DH), detrusor sphincter dyssynergia (DSD)	With neurologic lesion such as stroke, supraspinal cord lesion, multiple sclerosis	Simple cystometry or multichannel
	Detrusor hyperactivity with impaired contractility (DHIC)	Elderly, usually also associated with obstructive or stress symptoms	Multichannel CMG with or without EMG Videourodynamics
Stress	Hypermobility of bladder neck (female)	Detachment of bladder neck with concomitant hypermobility of the urethra.	Provocative stress test (direct visualization) Tests for bladder neck hypermobility Simple or multichannel CMG (to exclude DI) UPP or leak point pressure Videourodynamics
	Intrinsic sphincter deficiency (ISD)	Postoperative (after prostatectomy or anti-incontinence surgery), trauma, aging, radiation, congenital (epispadias)	Same as above
	Neurogenic sphincter deficiency	Neurogenic, sacral, or infrasacral lesion (e.g., myelomeningocele)	Same as above EMG
Overflow	Overflow from underactive or acontractile detrusor	Neurogenic (low spinal cord lesion, neuropathy, postradical pelvic surgery), idiopathic detrusor failure	Elevated PVR volume Uroflowmetry Voiding CMG (pressure flow) with EMG Cystourethroscopy
	Overflow from outlet obstruction	Male: prostate gland disease, urethral stricture Female: postoperative	Same as above Videourodynamics

[a] The urodynamic tests listed here are not recommended for routine use but are options for patients who require further evaluation (see text and Table 2). For details on various tests, see text. CMG = cystometrogram, EMG = electromyogram, PVR = postvoid residual, UPP = urethral pressure profilometry.

Urodynamic Tests. These tests are designed to determine the anatomic and functional status of the urinary bladder and urethra. The tests are performed by qualified professionals trained in the specific definitions and procedures.

In the further evaluation of UI, simple cystometry is appropriate for detecting abnormalities of detrusor compliance and contractability, measuring PVR, and determining capacity. (Strength of Evidence = A.)

In some instances of complicated diagnostic situations or involved therapeutic plans, multichannel cystometric tests are appropriate. (Strength of Evidence = B.)

When performing urodynamic studies, the health care provider should attempt to reproduce the patient's symptoms. (Strength of Evidence = C.)

No published research supports a need for cystometric testing in routine or basic evaluation of UI. However, cystometric tests remain important in certain clinical conditions, such as the ones delineated in Table 4.

Cystometry is a test of detrusor function. Depending on the technique used, cystometry can be used to assess bladder sensation, capacity, and compliance, and to determine the presence and magnitude of both voluntary and involuntary detrusor contractions. The patient's symptoms should be reproduced at the time of cystometry, because involuntary DI may be observed in asymptomatic patients and symptomatic patients may show no evidence of involuntary ventrusial contractions. On the other hand, cystometry may be falsely negative in a patient with a genuinely overactive bladder (McGuire, 1994). This is caused by heightened psychological inhibition of reflex activity or lack of measurable increase of detrusor pressure, urethral pressure, or electromyographic activity, which may be dissipated by poor urethral resistance and must therefore be examined closely.

Simple cystometry can be used to detect detrusor contractions and abnormalities of bladder compliance, and to measure PVR and determine bladder capacity (Ouslander, Leach, and Staskin, 1989; Sand, Brubaker, and Novak, 1991). This procedure is performed by filling the bladder to capacity by means of a urethral catheter. Because a rectal or vaginal catheter is not used to monitor the abdominal pressure, results must be interpreted with caution, especially in uncooperative or demented patients. Compared with multichannel studies, simple cystometry has a reported 75–100 percent sensitivity, 69–89 percent specificity, and 74–91 percent positive predictive value for the diagnosis of DI (Fonda, Brimage, and D'Astoli, 1993; Sand, Brubaker, and Novak, 1991; Sutherst and Brown, 1984).

A multichannel or subtracted cystometrogram (CMG) with simultaneous measurement of intra-abdominal, total bladder, and true detrusor pressures can differentiate an involuntary detrusor contraction or deversed bladder compliance from an increase in intra-abdominal pressure. However, few data are available comparing multichannel cystometrics with other measures of intravesical pressure, and it is suspected that false positives may be a problem, especially in elderly populations (Diokno, Brown, Brock, et al., 1988). Likewise, ambulatory continuous monitoring may reveal detrusor contractions missed during a provocative subtracted CMG (McGuire, 1994).

A voiding CMG or pressure flow study can measure detrusor contractility and detect outlet obstruction if the patient is able to void. Simultaneous measurement of detrusor and urethral pressures during voiding is especially helpful in diagnosing urodynamic obstruction (Diokno, 1990).

Uroflowmetry measures the urine flow rate visually, electronically, or with the use of a disposable unit. An electronically generated flow curve is considered helpful in identifying abnormal voiding patterns. Uroflowmetry is not helpful in diagnosing the types of incontinence found in women (Diokno, Normolle, Brown, et al., 1990; Fantl, Smith, Schneider, et al., 1983), but it may be helpful in patients who have difficulty with bladder emptying. However, this test cannot distinguish between obstruction and detrusor weakness without a simultaneous measurement of detrusor function.

Urethral pressure profilometry (UPP). The urethral function test measures resting and dynamic pressures in the urethra. Passive measurement of urethral pressures has been used by some investigators to help identify ISD, especially in women who have had previous operations. However, no specific measurement to date has been found to be discriminatory, especially in the elderly because of the normal decline of urethral pressures with age (Diokno, Normolle, Brown, et al., 1990). Dynamic measurements of urethral and bladder pressures may be used to measure the effect of exertion on the urethral closure mechanism. Sphincter function can also be assessed by measuring the abdominal or vesical pressure needed to overcome the urethral resistance (McGuire, Fitzpatrick, Wan, et al., 1993; McGuire, Woodside, Borden, et al., 1981; Wan, McGuire, Bloom, et al., 1993). The relative usefulness of the UPP versus that of Abdominal Leak Point Pressure (ALPP) has not been adequately studied.

Electromyography (EMG) of the striated urethral sphincter measures the integrity and function of its innervation. Both needle and surface EMG, in conjunction with CMG, may be helpful in diagnosing DSD (Diokno, Koff, and Anderson, 1976). However, this condition should be diagnosed only after common artifacts such as volitional tightening of the sphincter during involuntary detrusor contraction are excluded.

Endoscopic Tests

Cystoscopy is not recommended in the basic evaluation of UI. (Strength of Evidence = B.) However, cystoscopy may be indicated in the further evaluation when the following situations are present:

(a) sterile hematuria or pyuria (Strength of Evidence = B);

(b) when urodynamics fail to duplicate symptoms (Strength of Evidence = C);

(c) new onset of irritative voiding symptoms, bladder pain, recurrent cystitis, or suspected foreign body. (Strength of Evidence = B.)

Cystourethroscopy is a procedure that may help in identifying bladder lesions and foreign bodies, as well as urethral diverticula, fistula, strictures, or ISD. Most experts agree that cystoscopy is indicated for the evaluation of incontinent patients who have sterile hematuria or pyuria; recent (weeks to months) onset of irritative voiding symptoms such as frequency, urgency, and urge incontinence in the absence of any reversible causes (see Table 2); bladder pain; recurrent cystitis; or suspected intravesical foreign body; and when urodynamics fail to duplicate symptoms of UI.

A literature search revealed that in studies involving more than 600 incontinent patients selectively cystoscoped, only 11 (less than 2 percent) metaplastic or neoplastic lesions were identified (Awad, Gajewski, Katz, et al., 1992; Benson, 1985; Fischer-Rasmussen, Hansen, and Stage, 1986; Ouslander, Hepps, Raz, et al., 1986; Ouslander, Leach, Staskin, et al., 1989; Vehkalahti, Kivela, and Seppanen, 1986). Even in elderly, incontinent populations, the yield from selected cystoscopy is less than 1 percent (Ouslander, Hepps, Raz, et al., 1986). Therefore, cystoscopy should not be performed routinely in incontinent patients to exclude neoplasm.

The precise role of cystoscopy in the evaluation of incontinent patients is controversial. Data are scarce in the literature on this issue, and studies have a referral bias. Furthermore, urethroscopy is not as useful as urodynamic tests in diagnosing SUI (Scotti and Ostergard, 1993). Because this test is not performed during voiding, its usefulness in corroborating or excluding outlet obstruction is limited. Given the large numbers of patients with UI, and given the fact that the majority of UI patients are currently not cystoscoped, cystoscopy cannot be recommended as part of the routine evaluation until data are available to support its performance (Ouslander, Leach, and Staskin, 1989; Fischer-Rasmussen, Hansen, and Stage 1986).

Imaging Tests

Radiographic, ultrasonographic, and other imaging tests should be used for the evaluation of anatomic conditions associated with UI when clinically needed. (Strength of Evidence = C.)

Upper tract imaging is not a routine test to evaluate UI. Ultrasound of the kidneys, bladder, or both can help identify dilation of the upper urinary tract and renal pathology, especially in patients with urinary retention, abnormal renal function, or poorly compliant bladders. Excretory urography (i.e., intravenous pyelography) or other imaging modalities are indicated for incontinent patients with sterile hematuria or for further evaluation of upper tract obstruction or other pathology identified by ultrasound (Kumar and Schreib, 1985).

Lower tract imaging with and without voiding is helpful in examining the anatomy of the urinary bladder and urethra. Nonvoiding lateral cystourethrography in the resting and straining view can identify mobility or fixation of the bladder neck, funneling of the bladder neck and proximal urethra, and degree of cystocele. The voiding component can identify a urethral diverticulum, obstruction, and vesicoureteral reflux. Ultrasonography for assessing the dynamics of the bladder neck and urethra is still under investigation, and its clinical utility remains to be confirmed (Benson and Sumners, 1990; Mouritsen, Standberg, Jensen, et al., 1993; Quinn, Beynon, Mortensen, et al., 1988; Richmond and Sutherst, 1989b).

Videourodynamics is a technique that combines the various urodynamic tests with simultaneous fluoroscopy. The technique is helpful in sorting out causes of complex incontinence problems.

3 Treatment of Urinary Incontinence

The three major categories of treatment are

- Behavioral.

- Pharmacologic.

- Surgical.

Treatment options including their risks, benefits, and outcomes should be discussed with the patient so that informed choices can be made. As a general rule, the first choice should be the least invasive treatment with the fewest potential adverse complications that is appropriate for the patient. For many forms of UI, behavioral techniques meet these criteria. However, an informed patient's preference must be respected. A combination of surgical, behavioral, and pharmacologic interventions may be appropriate, but more research is required to determine the optimum treatment combinations for specific patient groups.

The role of other measures and supportive devices used in the management or treatment of UI is considered at the end of this chapter.

Behavioral Techniques

Behavioral techniques decrease the frequency of UI in most individuals when provided by knowledgeable health care providers, have no reported side effects, and do not limit future treatment options. Behavioral therapies can be divided into (1) caregiver-dependent techniques for patients with cognitive and motor deficits and (2) those requiring active rehabilitation and education techniques. These distinctions are arbitrary, however, and any individual's ability to actively participate varies on a continuum from complete dependence to full participation in the most complex behavioral therapies. For example, physically impaired patients who are cognitively intact may benefit from bladder training, pelvic muscle exercises (PMEs), and biofeedback therapy, but may depend on caregivers for assistance to the toilet.

Behavioral techniques are listed below in the order of those requiring passive involvement to those requiring active participation:

- Toileting assistance—routine/scheduled toileting, habit training, and prompted voiding.

- Bladder retraining.

- Pelvic muscle rehabilitation—PMEs, PMEs and bladder inhibition augmented by biofeedback therapy, PMEs augmented with vaginal weight training, and pelvic floor electrical stimulation.

All behavioral techniques involve educating the patient, the caregiver, or both, and provide positive reinforcement for effort and progress. Behavioral techniques should be offered to motivated individuals who wish to avoid more invasive procedures or dependence on protective garments, external devices, and medications. Behavioral techniques have few reported side effects and do not limit future treatment options. Behavioral techniques can increase patient understanding of lower urinary tract function and the environmental factors affecting symptoms. These techniques can improve control of detrusor and pelvic muscle function. They generally require patient or caregiver involvement and continued practice. If motivated, most people treated with behavioral techniques show improvement ranging from complete dryness to decreased incontinence episodes. Improved bladder control can occur even in the cognitively impaired individual (Colling, Ouslander, Hadley, et al., 1992; Engel, Burgio, McCormick, et al., 1990; McCormick, Cella, Scheve, et al., 1990; Schnelle, 1990). Behavioral techniques can also be used in combination with other therapies for UI.

Published results indicate that determining the precise level of effectiveness of behavioral interventions is limited by the following factors:

- Use of different outcome criteria.

- Variability in number, duration, and frequency of and adherence to treatment sessions.

- Variability of comprehensiveness in training procedures.

- Absence or variability in followup data.

- Concurrent application of multiple interventions that confound outcomes.

- Unspecified criteria for group assignment.

- Use of heterogeneous samples.

- Lack of measurement of independent variables.

- Uncontrolled inclusion of patients who had failed previous incontinence treatments.

- Lack of standardized terminology for the various behavioral techniques. (Because of the lack of standardized terminology, the reader must examine each study carefully and be alert to differences even in studies that appear to use the same terms.)

In general, however, studies show that behavioral interventions are effective in reducing incontinence. The cost of behavioral treatments compared with other treatments has not been studied, but two reports showed that the behavioral techniques enabled a considerable number of patients to avoid or postpone surgery (Cammu, Van Nylen, Derde, et al., 1991; Mouritsen, Frimodt, and Moller, 1991).

Assessment Before Behavioral Intervention

Before implementing behavioral therapy, patients should undergo the basic evaluation. Behavioral approaches must be tailored to the patient's underlying problem, such as bladder training or habit training for urge UI and pelvic muscle rehabilitation for SUI. Patients with overflow UI are not primary candidates for behavioral intervention.

Toileting Assistance

Toileting assistance interventions include routine or scheduled toileting, habit training, and prompted voiding.

Routine or scheduled toileting should be offered to incontinent patients on a consistent schedule. This technique is recommended for patients who cannot participate in independent toileting. (Strength of Evidence = C.)

Routine or scheduled toileting is provided by the caregiver on a fixed schedule at regular intervals. The caregiver takes the patient to void every 2–4 hours including at night. The goal is to keep the patient dry. No systematic effort is made to motivate the patient to delay voiding and resist urge, unlike in bladder retraining. In an uncontrolled, descriptive study of 161 male institutionalized patients, 20 patients who received a 4-week regimen of toileting every 2 hours eight times per day experienced an 85-percent improvement and were incontinent less than 20 percent of the time (Sogbein and Awad, 1982). In an uncontrolled, descriptive study of 20 females aged 24–94 years who were instructed to void every 2 hours regardless of urge for a period of 2 weeks, patients reported a 79-percent success rate (Godec, 1994). Burgio, Stutzman, and Engel (1989) studied 20 men postprostatectomy who followed a 2-hour voiding program for 2 weeks and reported a 33-percent increase in urgency, 29-percent decrease in stress UI, and no change in continual leakage.

Habit training is recommended for patients for whom a natural voiding pattern can be determined. (Strength of Evidence = B.)

Habit training is toileting scheduled to match the patient's voiding habits. One controlled study of habit training identified voiding patterns of 51 nursing home residents with an electronic monitoring device (Colling, Ouslander, Hadley, et al., 1992). The nursing home staff were taught to toilet the residents during the periods of greatest voiding frequency based on individual patterns identified by monitoring. A significant reduction in UI occurred during the 3-month intervention in 86 percent of the subjects, with one-third of this group showing 25 percent or greater improvement over baseline compared with an increase in UI observed in the control group. In addition, the volume of urine loss decreased significantly in the experimental group only. No side effects of habit training were reported. Nursing staff compliance was a problem, however, because of resistance to changes in care routines.

Habit training is an excellent technique for patients in the home living with a caregiver.

Prompted voiding is recommended in patients who can learn to recognize some degree of bladder fullness or the need to void, or who can ask for assistance or respond when prompted to toilet. Patients who are appropriate for prompted voiding may not have sufficient cognitive ability to participate in other, more complex behavioral therapies. (Strength of Evidence = A.)

The three major elements of prompted voiding are as follows:

- Monitoring—The patient is checked by caregivers on a regular basis and asked to report verbally if wet or dry.

- Prompting—The patient is asked (prompted) to try to use the toilet.

- Praising—The patient is praised for maintaining continence and for trying to toilet.

Prompted voiding has been shown to be effective in dependent or cognitively impaired nursing home incontinent patients (Schnelle, 1990; Hu, Igou, Kaltreider, et al., 1989; Burgio, McCormick, Scheve, et al., 1994; McCormick, Burgio, Engel, et al., 1992). Used as a supplement to habit training, prompted voiding reinforces discrimination of continence status, the need to urinate, and requests for toileting assistance from caregivers.

Four clinical trials, three controlled (Creason, Grybowski, Burgener, et al., 1989; Hu, Igou, Kaltreider, et al., 1989; Schnelle, 1990) and one uncontrolled (Burgio, McCormick, Scheve, et al., 1994), evaluated prompted voiding in nursing homes. The combined trials used prompted voiding for 251 residents and demonstrated significant reductions in incontinence with no reported side effects. An average reduction of 0.8–1.8 incontinence episodes per patient per day was reported. In contrast, the baseline number of incontinence episodes in control group subjects of approximately 4.5 times per 12-hour period remained unchanged over the course of the clinical trial. Residents with lower voiding frequencies (less than four in a 12-hour period) and those who toileted appropriately more than 75 percent of the time during a brief 2- to 6-day prompted voiding trial were the most likely to show long-term benefits with prompted voiding.

A clinical trial in seven nursing homes reported that nursing staff were able to maintain improved resident continence levels for 6 months in 76 residents who were identified as highly responsive to prompted voiding (Schnelle, Newman, White, et al., 1993). An earlier study showed that the behavioral training resulted in an estimated 76¢ savings per day per patient, and the investigators recommended that such training be instituted early after admission to maximize savings (Schnelle, Sowell, Hu, et al., 1988). Because nursing home staff administer the prompted voiding and habit training protocols, program success relies on training, compliance, and incentives for active staff participation. A 3-hour prompted voiding schedule can improve dryness in residents with mild to moderate UI (Burgio, McCormick, Scheve, et al., 1994).

Bladder Training

Bladder training is strongly recommended for management of urge (DI) and mixed incontinence. Bladder training is also recommended for management of SUI. (Strength of Evidence = A.)

Bladder training (also termed "bladder retraining") has many variations but generally consists of three primary components:

- Education.

- Scheduled voiding with systematic delay of voiding.

- Positive reinforcement.

The education program usually combines written, visual, and verbal instruction that addresses the physiology and pathophysiology of the lower urinary tract. A bladder training program requires the patient to resist or inhibit the sensation of urgency, to postpone voiding, and to urinate according to a timetable rather than according to the urinary urge (McCormick and Burgio, 1984). Bladder training may involve tactics that help distend the bladder, such as adjustment in fluid loads and delayed voiding to provide progressively larger voiding volumes and longer intervals between voids (Keating, Schulte, and Miller, 1988).

Initially, the interval goal is usually set between 2 and 3 hours or determined by the patient's present interval, and is not enforced during sleeping hours. The voiding schedule progressively increases the interval between mandatory voids with concomitant distraction or relaxation techniques. The patient is thus taught to delay voiding when the urge to void occurs. If the patient is unable to delay voiding between scheduled toileting times, the schedule is adjusted and the interval time is reset from the time of the last void. Another method is to keep the prearranged schedule and disregard the unscheduled void between schedules. The training may continue for several months, during which time the therapist provides positive reinforcement and instruction.

Bladder training has been used primarily to manage UI caused by DI. This form of training has few side effects but is difficult to implement in cognitively impaired persons. It may not be successful in frail, elderly patients.

Several reports demonstrate that bladder training is effective in reducing UI (Fantl, Wyman, McClish, et al., 1991; Ferrie, Smith, Logan, et al., 1984; Pengelly and Booth, 1980). Fantl, Wyman, McClish, et al. (1991) conducted a controlled, randomized study of 131 women with sphincteric incompetence and unstable detrusor function, 123 of whom had some followup data. Subjects receiving treatment participated in a bladder training program that included behavioral strategies to decrease urge, patient education, and a schedule of voiding. Of the 60 women in the treatment group, 12 percent became dry and 75 percent had at least a 50-percent reduction in the number of incontinent episodes. The magnitude of the effect was somewhat larger in the women with DI. The effect of bladder training was maintained after 6 months. Control subjects did not have significant changes in incontinent episodes. To date, no urodynamic variable has been shown to relate directly to the observed beneficial clinical effects.

Pelvic Muscle Rehabilitation

PMEs may be used alone or augmented with bladder inhibition biofeedback therapy or with vaginal weight training. Pelvic floor electrical stimulation is another method of pelvic muscle rehabilitation. Health care providers must teach patients the correct method of distinguishing and contracting the pelvic muscles through digital vaginal examination to verify appropriate muscle use, verbal feedback, or use of vaginal weights and biofeedback therapy to ensure accurate performance (Benvenuti, Caputo, Bandinelli, et al., 1987; Bump, Hurt, Fantl, et al., 1991; Burns, Marecki, Dittmar, et al., 1985; Dougherty, Abrams, and McKey, 1986; Keating, Schulte, and Miller, 1988).

Pelvic Muscle Exercise

Teaching women PMEs may prevent UI. (Strength of Evidence = C.)

Teaching exercises to strengthen pelvic muscles may decrease the incidence of UI. (Strength of Evidence = C.)

PMEs are strongly recommended for women with SUI. (Strength of Evidence = A.)

PMEs are also recommended in men and women in conjunction with bladder training for urge incontinence. (Strength of Evidence = B.)

PMEs may also benefit men who develop urinary incontinence following prostatectomy (Strength of Evidence = C.)

PMEs, also called Kegel exercises and pelvic floor exercises, are performed to strengthen the voluntary periurethral and perivaginal muscles (i.e., voluntary urinary sphincters and levator ani) that contribute to the closing force of the urethra and to the support of the pelvic visceral structures.

The first step in pelvic muscle re-education is to establish better awareness of pelvic muscle function. PMEs are performed by "drawing in" or "lifting up" of the perivaginal muscles and anal sphincter as if to control urination or defecation with minimal contraction of abdominal, buttock, or inner thigh muscles (Rose, Baigis-Smith, Smith, et al., 1990). Patients are generally told to sustain a contraction for at least 10 seconds, followed by an equal period of relaxation. The exercises should be performed about 30–80 times a day for at least 8 weeks and may need to be continued indefinitely. Elderly patients may require a longer time to train. In general, an individualized program of exercises and repetitions should be tailored to enhance muscle strength progressively (Ferguson, McKey, Bishop, et al., 1990). To condition the muscle to contract with increases in intra-abdominal pressure, patients should be taught to contract the pelvic muscles before and during situations when leakage may occur.

The specific effects of PMEs on actual lower urinary muscle function is not completely understood; some studies show a relationship between changes in various measures of pelvic floor strength, such as anal sphincter strength or maximum urethral closure pressure, and reduction in incontinence (Benvenuti, Caputo, Bandinelli, et al., 1987; Bo, Hagen, Kvarstein, et al., 1990; Ferguson, McKey, Bishop, et al., 1990; Dougherty, Bishop, Mooney, et al., 1993).

PMEs are indicated for women with stress incontinence and can reduce urgency and prevent urge UI (Burgio and Engel, 1990; Burgio, Robinson, and Engel, 1986; Burgio, Stutzman, and Engel, 1989; Burton, Pearce, Burgio, et al., 1988; Castleden, Duffin, Asher, et al., 1985; Klarskov, Nielsen, Kromman-Andersen, et al., 1991; McDowell, Burgio, Dombrowski, et al., 1992). They may be effective in reducing incontinence following prostatic surgery in men, but to date have only been tested for postprostatectomy in conjunction with a biofeedback component (Burgio, Stutzman, and Engel, 1989). PMEs are effective in reducing UI even after multiple surgical repairs in women (Baigis-Smith, Smith, Rose, et al., 1989; Brink, Wells, and Diokno, 1987; Burgio and Engel, 1990; Castleden, Duffin, and Mitchell, 1984; Ferguson, McKey, Bishop, et al., 1990; Heller, Whitehead, and Johnson, 1989; Henalla, Kirwan, Castleden, et al., 1988; Pearson and Droessler, 1988; Rose, Baigis-Smith, Smith, et al., 1990; Stoddart, 1983).

The effects of PME alone have been well documented in the medical literature. A summary of outcome findings from well-conducted studies follows.

Dougherty, Bishop, Mooney, et al. (1993) studied 65 women 35–75 years of age (mean age 51.3) and obtained a 62-percent reduction in UI episodes, and Ferguson, McKey, Bishop, et al. (1990) studied 20 women and demonstrated a 56- to 58-percent reduction in leakage as measured by 24-hour pad test using audiotape instruction in PME. Telephone contact and ongoing use of a bladder record may have contributed to the greater success found in these studies compared with others using a one-time instruction session.

To date, the most effective use of PME has been reported in an uncontrolled study by Benvenuti, Caputo, Bandinelli, et al. (1987), who provided 20 sessions of PME and other behavioral strategies and an intensive home program for a total of 10 contact hours to 20 women aged 35–65 years (mean age 50.8). In addition to a 95-percent reduction in incontinent episodes, significant changes were also reported FUL and MUCP at rest and during maximal voluntary contraction. A significant clinical benefit was consistent with changes in several physical measures of bladder function.

In a randomized clinical trial comparing PME and phenylpropanolamine hydrochloride (PPA), PME was found to be an effective alternative treatment for SUI comparable to PPA (Wells, Brink, Diokno, et al., 1991). Of the 54 subjects who completed the exercise program and the 64 who completed the drug protocol, 77 percent of the exercise subjects and 84 percent of the drug subjects reported improvement. The PME protocol involved 6 months of active PME taught with only written instruction, followed by monthly monitoring visits. The PPA was administered in doses of 50 mg daily for 2 weeks, increasing to twice daily if wetting continued. Adherence to the drug treatment was greater than to the exercise protocol.

Indications are that the intensity of the exercise program affects physiological and functional outcomes. Bo, Hagen, Kvarstein, et al. (1990) found that 52 subjects of mean age 45.9 years (range 24–64), randomized into a group receiving ongoing guidance in performing maximum contractions of the pelvic muscle that increased in intensity over 6 months, reported significantly greater reduction in incontinence and changes in physiological measures of pelvic floor strength compared with a group that received only a single session of instruction and a home exercise program. The group receiving the ongoing instruction reported a 60.1-percent cure/improvement rate compared with 17.3 percent attained in the home exercise group. This work also indicates a possible systematic relationship between symptom reduction and objective physical changes. Based on the data presented (Benvenuti, Caputo, Bandinelli, et al., 1987; Elia and Bergman, 1993; Mouritsen, Frimodt, and Moller, 1991), there is evidence that pelvic muscle re-education has the potential to change muscle physiology. Standards for assessment of change in pelvic muscle function have yet to be established, however.

PME also appears to be effective in the treatment of older adults. Flynn, Cell, and Luisi (1994) provided treatment for transient UI in 37 older adults receiving home nursing care (mean age 76) and behavioral strategies that included education in the maintenance of bowel regularity, bladder and habit training, fluid intake management, and PME. An 82.4-percent decrease in UI was attained with an average of five nursing visits. Because those patients with transient UI were not separated in the final analysis, the specific effect of the behavioral treatment is difficult to determine. Nonetheless, this report and others (Scheve, Engel, McCormick, et al., 1991) demonstrate the overall effectiveness of a well-directed nursing program, which includes PME for UI in homebound and long-term chronically ill patients.

Summary of findings. Evidence demonstrates that patients require repeated guidance over an extended period of time to derive optimal benefit from PME. Kegel himself recommended that patients be seen weekly to ensure that the exercises were being performed correctly. Further controlled studies are needed to demonstrate the most efficient method of teaching PME, exercise prescription, and the conditions in which biofeedback provides an added benefit to PME alone. It should also be noted that the majority of the research on PME is in women only.

PME and Bladder Inhibition Augmented by Biofeedback Therapy

Pelvic muscle rehabilitation and bladder inhibition using biofeedback therapy are recommended for patients with stress UI, urge UI, and mixed UI. (Strength of Evidence = A.)

Some type of biofeedback device is often used to assist patients to gain function and pelvic muscle awareness (Burns, Pranikoff, Nochajski, et al., 1990). The aim of biofeedback therapy, which uses electronic or mechanical instruments to relay information to patients about their physiologic activity, is to improve bladder dysfunction by teaching people to change physiologic responses that mediate bladder control (Burgio and Engel, 1990). Auditory or visual display of this information forms the core of biofeedback procedures (Schwartz, 1995). Biofeedback for UI typically uses single measurement (surface, needle, vaginal, or anal probe) EMG or manometric methods. Biofeedback using multimeasurement feedback methods involves simultaneous measurement of pelvic and abdominal/detrusor muscle activity. Biofeedback should be used in conjunction with other behavioral techniques such as PME and bladder training. As with all of the behavioral techniques, successful application of biofeedback depends greatly on the knowledge and skill of the health care provider, whose knowledge must include familiarity with evaluation techniques, anatomic and physiologic correlates of the different forms and symptoms of bladder dysfunction, instrumentation, and behavioral principles that guide the procedure.

Studies on the various applications of biofeedback combined with behavioral treatment report a range of 54–87 percent improvement in incontinence across various patient groups using different biofeedback and behavioral procedures. Some biofeedback protocols use only one measure for reinforcement of pelvic muscle contraction, whereas others use up to three, and include measures of abdominal and detrusor activity. The biofeedback protocol that has been associated with the largest and most consistent symptom reduction is one that reinforces pelvic muscle contraction concurrently with inhibition of abdominal and detrusor contraction. Reports using this multimeasurement method show a 75.9–82 percent reduction in UI across six studies involving 166 subjects (Burgio, Robinson, and Engel, 1986; Burgio, Stutzman, and Engel, 1989; Burgio, Whitehead, and Engel, 1985; Burton, Pearce, Burgio, et al., 1988; McDowell, Burgio, Dombrowski, et al., 1992). The presumed benefit of the multimeasurement procedure is that it reinforces pelvic floor contraction directly with moment-to-moment feedback, which characterizes for the patient the quality and intensity of the contraction. Without biofeedback, weak pelvic muscles may provide limited kinesthetic feedback to the desired contraction, and as a result the patient uses an attenuated internal reference to upgrade muscle contractions. Combining bladder and sphincter biofeedback also allows teaching pelvic muscle contraction in response to increasing bladder volume and observed detrusor activity.

In a controlled study, Burgio, Robinson, and Engel (1986) found that 13 subjects (mean age 47.9) receiving multimeasurement biofeedback reduced incontinence by 75.9 percent compared with a 51-percent reduction obtained in 11 subjects (mean age 40.7) who received only verbal feedback and instruction for PME with digital palpation. The multimeasurement biofeedback method has also been used successfully in the treatment of UI in postprostatectomy patients with urge and intermittent stress incontinence (Burgio, Stutzman, and Engel, 1989). However, another study demonstrated that when subjects complained primarily of urge incontinence, no benefit was obtained with the addition of biofeedback to behavioral training and PME, which was provided by a well-trained clinician over an average of five clinic sessions (Burton, Pearce, Burgio, et al., 1988). The results of this study should be interpreted with caution, however, because the groups differed in severity before treatment.

Several studies have also demonstrated significant reductions in UI associated with neurologic disease and in the frail elderly using a combination of multimeasurement biofeedback and other behavioral techniques such as bladder training (McDowell, Engberg, Weber, et al., 1994; Middaugh, Whitehead, Burgio, et al., 1989; O'Donnell and Doyle, 1991). Because multimeasurement biofeedback can provide specific reinforcement for pelvic muscle contraction that is isolated from counterproductive abdominal contraction, it is assumed that awareness of pelvic muscle contraction can be achieved more efficiently than from vaginal palpation alone.

In contrast to multimeasurement methods, the reduction in number of pad changes per 24 hours ranged from 43 to 54 percent when single-measurement biofeedback is used, when excluding a subgroup who had received only one biofeedback session (Wilson, Faragher, Butler, et al., 1987). This improvement was attained in an approximate average of 11 sessions (0.5–1.5 hours each). Another study (Susset, Galea, and Read, 1990) used single-channel biofeedback over six weekly clinic visits and a home trainer with which the subjects practiced daily. These subjects demonstrated an 87-percent reduction of leakage on pad test, suggesting that a home training device may provide an added benefit to clinic biofeedback visits, especially when only single-channel biofeedback is used.

In a randomized controlled study, Burns, Pranifoff, Nochajski, et al. (1993) studied 135 women (age range 55–75 years) with primary stress incontinence in three groups. One group received PME, and another group received single-measurement EMG biofeedback to perivaginal contraction for 20 minutes per week. The two treatment groups demonstrated a 54- to 61-percent reduction in incontinent episodes, compared with a 6-percent reduction of incontinence in the control group, but no difference between the two treatment groups was found. The improvements were maintained over a 6-month followup, and patients with moderate-to-severe symptoms showed even more improvement in the posttreatment phase. This study demonstrated that PME reduces incontinence and provided evidence that symptom severity has a role in response.

Further research is needed to determine which biofeedback protocols ensure that optimal outcomes are achieved in individual conditions and what methods provide the most valid measures of pelvic muscle function. The multimeasurement biofeedback appears to produce greater reduction in incontinence compared with PME alone or single measurement biofeedback. It is not known, however, to what degree detrusor or intra-abdominal pressure biofeedback individually contributes to the outcomes reported.

Summary of findings. Overall, the literature indicates that PME and other behavioral strategies, with or without biofeedback, can "cure" or reduce incontinence. Maximum benefit is derived from any pelvic muscle rehabilitation and education program when ongoing reinforcement and guidance are provided. Also, the intensity of the exercise program seems to influence both functional and physiological outcomes, and multimeasurement biofeedback protocols seem to yield the greatest and most consistent reductions in UI (Bo, Hagen, Kvarstein, et al., 1990; Burgio, Robinson, and Engel, 1986; Elia and Bergman, 1993; McDowell, Burgio, Dombrowski, et al., 1992).

Pelvic Muscle Exercises Augmented with Vaginal Weight Training

Vaginal weight training is recommended for SUI in premenopausal women. (Strength of Evidence = B.)

Specially designed vaginal weights for strengthening the pelvic muscles can augment PME. The patient receives a set of vaginal weights of identical shape and volume but of increasing weight (20–100 grams). As part of a structured progressive resistive exercise program, women insert the weight intravaginally, with the tapered portion resting on the superior surface of the perineal muscle and attempt to retain it by contracting the pelvic muscles up to 15 minutes. The weight is worn while the patient is ambulatory, and the exercise is done twice daily. The hypothesized mechanism of action is that the sustained contraction required to retain the weight increases the strength of the pelvic muscles, and the weight is assumed to provide heightened proprioceptive feedback to desired pelvic muscle contraction.

Available literature on this technique includes observations made in premenopausal women with SUI. Initial observations from four studies including 103 premenopausal women indicate subjective "cure" or greatly improved status of 68–80 percent after 4–6 weeks of treatment (Bridges, Denning, Olah, et al., 1988; Olah, Bridges, Denning, et al., 1990; Peattie and Plevnik, 1988; Peattie, Plevnik, and Stanton, 1988; Wilson and Borland, 1990). Objective outcome measures included reduction of urine loss on pad test, improvement in ability to hold heavier weights intravaginally, increased pelvic muscle strength (perineometer), and significant reduction in incontinence episodes. There were minimal or no adverse reactions. However, in several studies, PMEs were performed at the same time.

Although vaginal weight training may be useful in the treatment of stress incontinence, issues of applicability to other populations, particularly postmenopausal women with pelvic organ prolapse or other comorbid conditions, must be evaluated in terms of treatment protocols and long-term effects.

Pelvic Floor Electrical Stimulation

Pelvic floor electrical stimulation has been shown to decrease incontinence in women with SUI. (Strength of Evidence = B.)

Pelvic floor electrical stimulation may be useful for urge and mixed incontinence. (Strength of Evidence = B.)

Pelvic floor electrical stimulation (nonimplantable) produces a contraction of the levator ani, external urethral and anal sphincters, accompanied by a reflex inhibition of the detrusor; this activity depends on a preserved reflex arc through the sacral micturition center (Vodusek, Plevnik, Vrtacnik, et al., 1988). Nonimplantable pelvic floor electrical stimulation uses vaginal or anal sensors or surface electrodes (Vodusek, Plevnik, Vrtacnik, et al., 1988). Adverse reactions are minimal and include pain and discomfort. Studies vary regarding the type and placement of electrodes; frequency, duration, and amplitude of voltage; and whether the stimulation was phasic, intermittent, or continuous. Several of these studies address long-term followup with reports that the effects for cured or improved patients ranged from 54 to 77 percent (Bent, Sand, Ostergard, et al., 1993; Bergmann and Eriksen, 1986; Blowman, Pickles, Emery, et al., 1991; Caputo, Bensen, McClellan, et al., 1993; Eriksen, 1990; Eriksen, Bergmann, and Mjolnerod, 1987; Eriksen, Bergmann, and Eik-Nes, 1989; Esa, Kiwamoto, Sugiyama, et al., 1991; Fall, Ahlstrom, Carlsson, et al., 1986; Fossberg, Sorensen, Ruutu, et al., 1990; Green and Laycock, 1990; Hahn, Sommar, and Fall, 1991; Lamhut, Jackson, and Wall, 1992; Leach and Bavendam, 1989; Lose, Andersen, and Kristensen, 1986; McIntosh, Frahm, Mallett, et al., 1993; Meyer, Dhenin, Schmidt, et al., 1992; Eriksen and Mjolnerod, 1987; Nakamura, Sakurai, Tsujimoto, et al., 1986; Nakamura, Sakurai, Sugao, et al., 1987; Ohlsson, Fall, and Frankenberg-Sommar, 1989; Plevnik, Joney, Vrtacnik, et al., 1986; Sand, Richardson, Staskin, et al., 1995; Wilson, 1990; Zollner-Nielsen and Samuelsson, 1992).

Two randomized controlled trials have been conducted. Using active and placebo perianal surface patch neurostimulation for SUI in patients, Blowman, Pickles, Emergy, et al. (1991) reported a "cure" or improvement rate of 86 percent in the active group ($N=7$) and 33 percent in the placebo group ($N=6$). Electrical stimulation was not used as a single therapy, however; both groups also received instruction in PME. Using active and inactive vaginal plug devices in 52 women with SUI, Sand, Richardson, Staskin, et al. (1995) reported objective "cure" or improvement in 48 percent of the active device group and in 13 percent of the placebo group. Active device patients had significant improvements in UI episodes, leakage volume, and vaginal muscle strength and in subjective improvement measures when compared with the placebo group.

In other studies with similar settings, anal or vaginal plug devices were used for maximal electrical stimulation for 4 weeks to 3.5 months, 20 minutes to 20 hours/day. "Cure" or improvement rates ranged from 48 to 94 percent in 842 patients with stress, urge, or mixed incontinence. The effects of therapy were sustained 6 weeks to 2 years in 54–77 percent of patients, especially if patients continued to do PME after treatment (Bergman and Eriksen, 1986; Blowman, Pickles, Emery, et al., 1991; Bridges, Denning, Olah, et al., 1988; Caputo, Bensen, McClellan, et al., 1993; Eriksen, Bergmann, and Eik-Nes, 1989; Eriksen, Bergmann, and Mjolnerod, 1987; Eriksen and Eik-Nes, 1989; Esa, Kiwamoto, Sugiyama, et al., 1991; Fossberg, Sorensen, Ruutu, et al., 1990; Kunkle, Payne, and Whitmore, 1993; Meyer, Dhenin, Schmidt, et al., 1992; Plevnik, Joney, Vrtacnik, et al., 1986; Sand, Richardson, Staskin, et al., 1995; Zollner-Nielsen and Samuelsson, 1992). One study of cognitively impaired patients in a nursing home showed no significant effect of stimulation, with a trend toward increased wetness (Lamhut, Jackson, and Wall, 1992).

Summary of findings. Research indicates that pelvic floor electrical stimulation can significantly reduce UI in women with SUI, and may be effective in men and women with mixed and urge UI. Stimulation may be effective when augmented with other pelvic muscle rehabilitation therapies. Minimal adverse side effects occur with this treatment. Treatment using stimulation requires monitoring by a health care provider to determine effectiveness. Further research is needed to determine the efficacy of pelvic floor stimulation used alone or in combination with other therapies. Standardization of the parameters of the techniques used, such as that proposed by the International Continence Society, is necessary to allow further comparison of study results.

Pharmacologic Treatment[a,b]

Several medications have proven to be beneficial for treating UI, although their risk-to-benefit ratios are difficult to gauge precisely because of deficiencies in study design. Some of the limitations of published trials include variable inclusion and exclusion criteria or inadequate (small) sample size; inconsistent definition of outcome criteria; short study durations; fixed drug dosages that may have been excessive or inadequate; analyses confounded by other interventions such as behavioral manipulations; and limited compliance data and nonuniform methods for collecting, reporting, and comparing side effects. Summarized below are data derived from randomized controlled trials of orally administered medications, vaginally administered medications, or both, used to treat UI. Recommendations pertaining to the benefits, risks, and utility of pharmacologic therapies are noted, including the strength of evidence.

---

[a] Of the pharmacologic treatments discussed in this chapter, only oxybutynin and flavoxate have been officially approved by the FDA for the indicated use. The remainder are not approved but are commonly used.

[b] Imipramine is officially approved by the FDA for enuresis in children but not adults.

Urge Incontinence: Detrusor Instability _______________________

The following pharmacologic agents are reported to be useful in DI as observed in clinical practice. (Strength of Evidence = B.)

- Anticholinergic agents: oxybutynin, dicyclomine hydrochloride, and propantheline.

- Tricyclic antidepressants: imipramine, doxepin, desipramine, and nortriptyline.

Anticholinergic Agents

Anticholinergic agents are the first-line pharmacologic therapy for patients with DI. (Strength of Evidence = A.)

When pharmacologic therapy is to be used for patients with DI, oxybutynin is the anticholinergic agent of choice. The recommended dosage is 2.5–5 mg taken orally three or four times per day. (Strength of Evidence = A.)

Propantheline is the second-line anticholinergic agent in the treatment of patients with DI who can tolerate the full dosage. The recommended dosages are 7.5–30 mg administered three to five times per day; higher dosages (15–60 mg qid) may be required. (Strength of Evidence = B.)

Flavoxate is not recommended for the treatment of patients with DI. (Strength of Evidence = A.)

Anticholinergic agents are effective as treatment for UI because they block contraction of the normal bladder and probably the unstable bladder as well. All anticholinergic drugs are contraindicated in patients with documented narrow-angle, but not wide-angle, glaucoma.

Oxybutynin has both anticholinergic and direct smooth muscle relaxant properties. Seven randomized controlled studies of the use of this agent for UI were identified. Oxybutynin proved superior to placebo in six studies of middle-aged outpatients, reducing incontinence frequency by 15–58 percent over the response to placebo (Holmes, Montz, and Stanton, 1989; Moore, Hay, Imrie, et al., 1990; Riva and Casolati, 1984; Tapp, Cardozo, Versi, et al., 1990; Thuroff, Bunke, Ebner, et al., 1991; Zeegers, Kiesswetter, Kramer, et al., 1987). In two of these studies, 43 percent and 67 percent of subjects became subjectively continent, a much better result than occurred with placebo (Moore, Hay, Imrie, et al., 1990; Riva and Casolati, 1984). Only one study reported a benefit with a dosage of 15 mg tid-qid (Holmes, Montz, and Stanton, 1989), whereas a second showed no improvement over placebo (Thuroff, Bunke, Ebner, et al., 1991). In the only trial that failed to note a benefit, oxybutynin was used less frequently (5 mg bid) in elderly nursing home residents (Zorzitto, Holliday, Jewett, et al., 1989). Oxbutynin has also been effective and well tolerated when instilled into the bladder of study patients, primary those with neuropathic bladder (Mizunaga, Miyata, Kaneko, et al., 1994).

Side effects were noted in all studies and included dry skin, blurred vision, change in mental status, nausea, constipation, and marked xerostomia (dry mouth). Severity increased with dosage, with severe xerostomia occurring in 84 percent of subjects receiving 5 mg of oxybutynin four times per day (Tapp, Cardozo, Versi, et al., 1990).

Propantheline is the prototype for anticholinergic agents used for urologic conditions. No agent better approximates atropine's effect on the bladder *in vitro*, although its central nervous system side effects are less marked. Moreover, propantheline is inexpensive and has been widely used over time.

Despite propantheline's success in uncontrolled case series, only five adequately controlled trials could be identified (Blaivas, Labib, Michalik, et al., 1980; Dequeker, 1965; Holmes, Montz, and Stanton, 1989; Thuroff, Burke, Ebner, et al., 1991; Zorzitto, Jewett, Fernie, et al., 1986), three of which included only elderly nursing home residents with advanced dementia. Only one study reported a benefit with a dosage of 15 mg tid-qid (Holmes, Montz, and Stanton, 1989). Two of the nursing home studies evaluated higher dosages of propantheline (30 mg qid; 15 mg tid + 60 mg at bedtime (hs)) and found that incontinence frequency was reduced by 13–17 percent over placebo—a small but statistically significant improvement in both studies (Dequeker, 1965; Zorzitto, Jewett, Fernie, et al., 1986). In one of these trials, side effects were reported in half of the subjects, one-fifth of whom withdrew because of severe side effects (Zorzitto, Jewett, Fernie, et al., 1986); no side effects were reported in the trial using the 60 mg hs dosage. In a dose titration study, dosages up to 60 mg qid were associated with complete response in 25 of 26 patients (Blaivas, Labib, Michalik, et al., 1980).

In addition to urinary retention, side effects associated with propantheline, as with all anticholinergic agents, include visual blurring, xerostomia, nausea, constipation, tachycardia, drowsiness, and confusion; the most common of these was xerostomia.

Despite the lack of adequate trials, consensus among experts is that at least for less impaired patients who can tolerate full dosages, propantheline is effective (Andersson, 1988; Wein, 1990).

Dicyclomine hydrochloride is an anticholinergic agent with smooth muscle relaxant properties. Studies on the use of this drug for UI are limited, and the populations that have been studied were small. One pilot trial and one larger randomized controlled trial were identified (Beck, Arnusch, and King, 1976; Castleden, Duffin, and Millar, 1987). In the larger study, 62 percent of subjects improved on dicyclomine 10 mg tid (90 percent of whom became continent) compared with 20 percent on placebo (65 percent of whom became continent); statistical significance was not specified, and side effects were not mentioned (Beck, Arnush, and King, 1976). Results were similar in the smaller pilot study (Castleton, Duffin, and Millar, 1987).

Studies comparing dicyclomine with other anticholinergic agents are not available. This agent may be used as an alternative treatment for UI, however, pending further research. The dosage is 10–20 mg taken orally three times daily.

Flavoxate is a tertiary amine that has demonstrated smooth muscle relaxant properties *in vitro*. Although flavoxate is widely used for incontinence, only four randomized controlled studies of its efficacy for UI could be identified (Meyhoff, Gerstenberg, and Nordling, 1983; Robinson and Brocklehurst, 1983; Zeegers, Kiesswetter, Kramer, et al., 1987; Chapple, Parkhouse, Gardener, et al., 1990). None demonstrated a significant benefit. At present, this drug is not recommended for the treatment of UI.

Hyoscyamine and other oral anticholinergics are known to be used in clinical practice in the treatment of DI; however, no scientific literature that met the panel's criteria addressed the use of these agents for patients with UI. The panel therefore is not making recommendations regarding these drugs.

Calcium Channel–Blocking Agents. Influx of extracellular calcium is important for detrusor muscle contraction and can be blocked by calcium channel antagonists. Although such agents are often advocated for bladder storage disorders, only a few small, but favorable, case series were identified in the literature. No controlled studies could be found for marketed agents (e.g., nifedipine, diltiazem, verapamil). One placebo-controlled study of flunarizine that showed a positive effect was identified; however, in a subsequent 1-month controlled trial by the same investigators, its efficacy diminished, and the high (but unreported) rate of side effects led the investigators to temper their original enthusiasm (Palmer, Worth, and Exton-Smith, 1981). At this time, these agents are not recommended for general use for the treatment of detrusor instability.

Terodiline. An investigational drug in the United States, terodiline possesses calcium channel–blocking and anticholinergic properties. It has demonstrated *in vivo* activity in the treatment of DI. However, recent reports of serious ventricular arrhythmias have resulted in its temporary removal from the European market and discontinuation of trials in the United States.

Tricyclic Agents

The use of tricyclic agents (TCAs) should be reserved for carefully evaluated patients. The usual oral dosages are 10–25 mg initially administered one to three times per day, but less frequent administration is usually possible because of the long half-life of these drugs. The daily total dosage is usually 25–100 mg. (Strength of Evidence = B.)

Although TCAs are widely used, they produce many adverse effects (e.g., cardiac and anticholinergic), with the risk more likely in elderly patients. Limited research on the use of TCAs is available. Only three randomized controlled studies were identified. One conducted with psychiatric inpatients in whom the type of UI was not established showed that imipramine, desipramine, and nortriptyline each resulted in a statistically significant reduction in the number of "wet nights" (Milner and Hills, 1968). Side effects were rare and minor except for paralytic ileus in one case.

The other two studies, one using doxepin (Lose, Jorgensen, and

Thunedborg, 1989) and the other imipramine (Castleden, Duffin, and Gulati, 1986), documented decreases in incontinence frequency. However, the results were statistically significant only for reducing nocturnal incontinence and overall patient preference for doxepin. Side effects in these studies included fatigue, xerostomia, dizziness, and blurred vision in the doxepin group and nausea and insomnia in the imipramine group.

Nonsteroidal Anti-Inflammatory Drugs

Nonsteroidal anti-inflammatory drugs (NSAIDs) are not recommended for the primary treatment of DI. (Strength of Evidence = C.)

NSAIDs are theorized to be effective for UI because of their inhibition of prostaglandin "synthetase," which interferes with prostaglandin-mediated bladder contractions. However, limited research on the use of NSAIDs for patients with UI is available. Two controlled trials in women have been conducted (Cardozo and Stanton, 1979; Cardozo, Stanton, Robinson, et al., 1980). In a non–placebo-controlled trial, patients receiving indomethacin 100 mg po bid experienced comparable resolution of UI compared with those receiving bromocriptine (Cardozo and Stanton, 1979). A placebo-controlled trial demonstrated 55-percent continence with flurbiprofen 50 mg po tid versus 29 percent with placebo (Cardozo, Stanton, Robinson, et al., 1980). In both studies, side effects were frequent, although no patient stopped use of NSAIDs. When NSAIDs are used, close monitoring for drug toxicity (e.g., gastrointestinal hemorrhage, renal dysfunction) should be performed, especially in elderly patients.

Other Drugs of Possible Benefit. Other drugs used for detrusor instability include a beta-adrenergic agonist (terbutaline) (Lindholm and Lose, 1986) and a spinal synaptic inhibitor (baclofen) (Taylor and Bates, 1979). Limited studies and clinical experience with these agents suggest that further studies must be done before they can be recommended for general use.

Summary of findings. Pharmacotherapy, at least in short-term trials, appears to benefit some patients with UI due to detrusor instability. However, regardless of the agent chosen, involuntary bladder contractions are usually not abolished, the "warning time" between appreciation of the need to void and the onset of bladder contraction is usually not affected, the degree of improvement is modest, and "cure" is uncommon. In addition, many of these medications are costly, and most have bothersome side effects. These drugs should be used only in conjunction with a voiding schedule or behavioral intervention and only after other factors contributing to incontinence have been addressed.

To date, oxybutynin possesses the most favorable efficacy, safety, and pharmacokinetics profile of the agents for DI. However, selection of an agent must be individualized and based on patient considerations (i.e., contraindications) and cost as well as on drug considerations (i.e., kinetics, drug interactions, and side effects). For example, an antidepressant may be the preferred drug for UI in a depressed patient but not for a patient with orthostatic hypotension who is prone to falling. A drug with a rapid onset of action may be useful for a patient who desires protection only for certain events (e.g., going out for the afternoon), whereas a drug with a longer half-life may be preferable for a patient who desires continuous protection.

Regardless of the agent selected, the initial dosage should be relatively low. The dosage should be increased slowly, consistent with the drug's half-life, and titrated to balance efficacy with side effects. Patients must be closely monitored for urinary retention. Combining agents with different mechanisms of action may increase their efficacy and reduce side effects, but few relevant data are available. Although the long-term efficacy of bladder relaxants is largely unknown, Moore, Hay, Imrie, et al. (1990) have reported that once incontinence responded to pharmacologic and behavioral interventions, improvement persisted even if the medication was withdrawn after a few months.

Stress Incontinence: Urethral Sphincter Insufficiency _____

The rationale for pharmacologic therapy for UI due to urethral sphincter insufficiency (stress incontinence, SUI) is based on selection of agents that affect the high concentration of alpha-adrenergic receptors in the bladder neck, bladder base, and proximal urethra. Sympathomimetic drugs with alpha-adrenergic agonist activity presumably cause muscle contraction in these areas and thereby increase bladder outlet resistance. Pharmacotherapeutic strategies that are designed to increase bladder outlet resistance include the use of drugs with direct alpha-adrenergic agonist activity, estrogen supplementation both for direct effect on urethral mucosal and periurethral tissues and for enhancement of alpha-adrenergic response, and beta-adrenergic-blocking drugs that may allow unopposed stimulation of alpha-receptor–mediated contractile muscle responses.

Alpha-Adrenergic Agonist Drugs

Phenylpropanolamine (PPA) or pseudoephedrine is the first-line pharmacologic therapy for women with SUI who have no contraindications for its use, particularly hypertension. The recommended dosage for PPA is 25–100 mg in sustained-release form, administered orally, twice daily. The usual dosage of pseudoephedrine is 15–30 mg, orally, three times daily. (Strength of Evidence = A.)

PPA in sustained-release form is the major alpha-adrenergic agonist drug studied in women with stress incontinence. Seven prospective randomized controlled studies of middle-aged, normotensive women with stress incontinence were reviewed. In three studies (Collste and Lindskog, 1987; Fossberg, Beisland, and Lundgren, 1983; Lehtonen, Rannikko, Lindell, et al., 1986) no patients became continent, but 31–45 percent of patients given PPA had decreased incontinence over placebo response (PPA minus placebo "improved" response). In four studies (Ek, Andersson, Gullberg, et al., 1978;

Hilton, Tweddell, and Mayne, 1990; Walter, Kjaergaard, Lose, et al., 1990; Wells, Brink, Diokno, et al., 1991), 9–14 percent of women became dry, and 19–60 percent of patients experienced significant reduction of incontinence over the number of similar responses in the placebo group. In studies in which the improvement rate was reported, the reduction in leakage with PPA ranged from 31 to 60 percent over the response with placebo.

Side effects were minimal and included nausea, xerostomia, insomnia, rash, itching, and restlessness. PPA did not cause significant increases in blood pressure during the evaluation period.

Summary of findings. Pharmacologic therapy of incontinence caused by sphincter insufficiency (stress incontinence) using PPA appears to result in few cures or dryness (0–14 percent) but may cause subjective improvement in 20–60 percent of patients over placebo response. It is unclear whether patient age or the severity of leakage affects the likelihood of response. Possible side effects from alpha-adrenergic agonist drugs include anxiety, insomnia, agitation, respiratory difficulty, headache, sweating, hypertension, and cardiac arrhythmias, all of which may occur more commonly in elderly patients. The risk of PPA use in hypertensive women and its efficacy in women taking antihypertensive drugs have not been determined. PPA should be used with caution in patients with hypertension, hyperthyroidism, cardiac arrhythmias, and angina. The sustained-release form is advocated because of its routine use by investigators in clinical trials. Whether the immediate-release form produces similar results has not been established.

Estrogen Therapy

Estrogen (oral or vaginal) may be considered as an adjunctive pharmacologic agent for postmenopausal women with SUI or mixed incontinence. Conjugated estrogen is usually administered either orally (0.3–1.25 mg/day) or vaginally (2 g or fraction/day). Progestin (e.g., medroxyprogesterone 2.5–10 mg/day) may be given continuously or intermittently. (Strength of Evidence = B.)

Because the vagina and urethra are of similar embryologic origin, estrogen supplementation in postmenopausal women may restore urethral mucosal coaptation and increase vascularity, tone, and the alpha-adrenergic responsiveness of urethral muscle, which in turn may increase bladder outlet resistance and decrease stress incontinence. However, the exact role of estrogen, as well as its mechanism of action, is still unknown and deserves further research. Most clinical trials have been conducted with estrogen products available abroad; but their data are included in this report because of the paucity of research using marketed products in the United States and the similarities between estrogens.

Estriol derivatives. Two studies of postmenopausal women with stress incontinence compared effects of placebo and estriol, 4 mg/day, on continence (Samsioe, Jansson, Mellstrom, et al., 1985; Walter, Kjaergaard, Lose, et al.,

1990). Results showed that 0–14 percent of patients on estriol became dry, and 29 percent of patients experienced improved continence compared with patients who received placebo. One study showed that the response to estriol was significantly better than to placebo (Walter, Kjaergaard, Lose, et al., 1990), whereas the other study showed that the response to active drug was not significantly better than to placebo (Samsioe, Jansson, Mellstrom, et al., 1985). In the latter study, 66 percent of patients with UI reported improvement.

A trial of quinestradol, an estriol derivative, in female incontinent nursing home residents did not result in continence, but 89 percent of patients had a significant reduction of leakage episodes while taking quinestradol compared with 0 percent while on placebo (Judge, 1969).

Estrone derivatives. A 3-month prospective study of postmenopausal stress-incontinent women who received placebo or piperazine estrone sulfate for 3 weeks with one drug-free week per cycle revealed that subjective and objective improvements at 3 months were greater, but not statistically significant, while on estrogen (Wilson, Faragher, Butler, et al., 1987).

Fantl, Cardozo, McClish, et al. (1994) provided a meta-analysis from 6 randomized controlled trials and 17 uncontrolled clinical series. Favorable effects on incontinence in postmenopausal women were found with estrogen therapy ($P < 0.01$ for all subjects and $P < 0.05$ for those with SUI).

Summary of findings. Limited evidence suggests that estrogen therapy by oral or vaginal administration may benefit some patients with SUI and mixed UI. Its effect on urge UI has not been reported in most of the available literature.

Other beneficial effects of long-term estrogen may include decreased risk of stroke, ischemic heart disease, and osteoporosis. Estrogen replacement should be given with a progestin when the uterus is present to avoid unopposed estrogen stimulation of the endometrium, particularly if prolonged therapy is anticipated. The dosages of estrogen and progestin used vary. Risks of estrogen therapy given in this manner include neoplasia of estrogen-responsive organs. Thus, estrogen therapy is contraindicated in patients with known or suspected cancer of the breast or uterus.

Alpha-Adrenergic Agonist and Estrogen Supplementation

Combination therapy of oral or vaginal estrogens and PPA is recommended in the treatment of SUI in postmenopausal women when initial single-drug therapy has proven inadequate. (Strength of Evidence = A.)

The rationale supporting combined estrogen supplementation and alpha-adrenergic agonist therapy in postmenopausal women with incontinence due to sphincteric insufficiency is based on an estrogen-induced increased number, sensitivity of alpha-adrenergic receptors in the urethra, or both, which potentiates the alpha-adrenergic contractile response to drug stimulation.

Review of four controlled studies that combined estrogen and alpha-adrenergic agonist therapy suggests that the combined therapy may be more effective than alpha-adrenergic agonist therapy alone (Ek, Andersson, Gullberg, et al., 1978, 1980; Hilton, Tweddell, and Mayne, 1990; Walter, Kjaergaard, Lose, et al., 1990). However, the studies are limited, and based on these results, combination therapy should be considered when initial single-drug therapy fails. The possible risks of alpha-adrenergic agonist drugs and estrogen do not appear to be increased when used together. Patients should be carefully monitored when combination therapy is prescribed, however.

Other Drugs of Possible Benefit

Imipramine is recommended as an alternative pharmacologic therapy for SUI when first-line agents have proven unsatisfactory. (Strength of Evidence = C.)

Imipramine. A tricyclic antidepressant that possesses both alpha-adrenergic agonist activity (presumably mediated by blocking reuptake of norepinephrine) and anticholinergic properties has been reported to benefit women with stress incontinence. In a nonrandomized, uncontrolled study, 30 women (28–64 years old) with pure stress incontinence received imipramine at 75 mg daily for 4 weeks; 21 of the 30 (70 percent) claimed continence (Gilja, Radej, Kovacic, et al., 1984). Side effects reported included nausea, insomnia, weakness, fatigue, and postural hypotension. Prospective controlled studies are not available, and thus further research is necessary.

The use of propranolol or other beta-blockers cannot be recommended for treatment of SUI because of lack of clinical experience and clinical studies. (Strength of Evidence = C.)

Propranolol. Limited research on the use of beta-blockers for treatment of SUI is available. In one uncontrolled study, a beta-adrenergic-blocking drug was reported to improve symptoms of SUI (Gleason, Reilly, Bottaccini, et al., 1974). The use of this and other beta-blockers cannot be recommended for treatment of incontinence at this time.

Antidiuretic hormone. Desmopressin (desmopressin diacetate arginine vasopressin (DDAVP)) is used mainly in the treatment of nocturnal enuresis and night-time polyuria. Available research on this drug has been conducted mainly in children and in patients with neuropathic conditions. Because few data exist in adults, DDAVP is not discussed in detail in this guideline.

Surgical Treatment

The decision to perform surgery for the treatment of UI should be made only after a precise, focused assessment that includes a comprehensive clinical evaluation with an objective confirmation of the pathophysiologic diagnosis and severity of urinary loss, a correlation of the anatomic and physiologic findings with the surgical plan, an estimation of surgical risk, and an estimation of the impact of the proposed surgery on the patient's quality of life.

Several caveats must be considered when reviewing the literature on the surgical treatment of UI. Standards have not been established for describing the patient population, the type of incontinence, the methods for accurate diagnosis, the techniques of the surgical procedure, or the outcome in different domains (e.g., symptoms, anatomophysiologic outcomes, quantity of fluid loss, quality of life). There may be difficulty in comparing surgical procedures because of intentional modifications or variations in technique and the experience and expertise of the surgeon. Postoperative reporting is often biased by variations in the definitions for failure, improvement, and success, and similarly for the degree and incidence of operative morbidity, early and late complications, and length of followup. These variations make precise comparisons of studies including different surgeons performing the same procedure, or multiple surgeons performing different procedures, impossible. Retrospective comparison of different techniques may contain unknown selection biases. Prospective comparisons often include different surgeons with different degrees of experience and expertise. Terminology should be standardized for classification of incontinence, description and execution of surgical procedures, and reporting of surgical outcomes. In reports of series, complications should be reported individually, and the criteria for patient selection should be described. Comparison of different techniques should be made by prospective randomized studies using similar inclusion criteria for each technique.

This guideline is primarily directed toward the primary care provider, and the level of detail provided is not sufficient to direct surgical therapy. The inherent variability in surgical technique and the way in which operations are performed make it impossible to direct surgical practice in a guideline of this scope.

The objectives of surgical treatment of incontinence depend on the specific etiology. A given patient may have more than one etiology. In this guideline, each etiology is addressed separately. The purpose of a surgical procedure is to correct, compensate for, or circumvent the underlying pathology causing urinary loss. Stress incontinence in women may be caused by urethral hypermobility or ISD. Men with stress incontinence suffer solely from ISD. Inappropriate elevations in bladder pressure may result from uninhibited bladder contractions or a loss of bladder compliance. Poor bladder emptying that leads to retention may result from an impaired or absent bladder contraction or from outlet obstruction.

The surgical procedures described in this section are divided into three sections: (1) surgeries that *increase outlet resistance* and relieve SUI and ISD, (2) procedures that *decrease detrusor instability* and correct urge incontinence, and (3) operations that *remove outlet obstruction*, thereby correcting overflow incontinence or reversing detrusor instability that is secondary to the outlet obstruction.

Surgery is recommended for treatment of stress incontinence in men and women and may be recommended as first-line treatment for appropriately selected patients who are unable to comply with other nonsurgical therapies. (Strength of Evidence = B.)

Stress Incontinence in Women:
Hypermobility or Intrinsic Sphincter Deficiency ___________

The surgical objective in cases of hypermobility is to improve the support of the sphincter unit without obstruction. On the other hand, the goal of surgery for ISD is to increase urethral coaptation and resistance. Although many operations result in both improved support and compression of the proximal urethra, a primarily supportive procedure is less likely to succeed for a patient with ISD than for a patient with only hypermobility.

Preoperative Evaluation. A preoperative evaluation is important to ensure proper patient selection and to determine the appropriate surgical procedure. The evaluation should include a comprehensive history, physical examination, urinalysis, urine culture, and measurement of PVR volume. It is important to document the incontinence objectively by direct observation of a positive stress test (direct visualization). Some multiparous women may have stress incontinence on physical examination but are not troubled by this; therefore, the patient should be asked if the incontinence visible on examination is the type of incontinence that led her to seek care. Because CMGs may be falsely negative in many women with DI, simply using a negative CMG to diagnose SUI is not acceptable. When further corroboration is needed, cystoscopy, a cystogram with straining, measurement of Valsalva leak point pressure, dynamic UPP, or a combination may be used.

Although patients with symptoms of DI may be more likely to remain incontinent after surgery, it is not clear whether a preoperative CMG to search for asymptomatic instability is necessary. If symptomatic instability is present, some health care providers may attempt behavioral or pharmacologic treatment before surgical correction of the stress incontinence. Others may not because many patients experience resolution of DI once stress incontinence is corrected. This decision must be made on an individual basis, using clinical judgment and considering the patient's informed preference.

To select the appropriate surgical procedure, one must assess the position of the urethra and the degree of axial urethral mobility by physical examination, cystogram, ultrasound, or cystoscopy. Factors that may be associated with an increased risk of failure, such as symptomatic DI, obesity, prior surgery, hypoestrogenism, chronic cough, strenuous physical activity, previous radiation therapy, advanced age, or poor nutrition, must be identified. Pelvic organ prolapse or other pathology that would require surgical treatment at the same time as the anti-incontinence procedure should also be identified. The approach required to treat the concurrent pathology will influence the choice of approach for the anti-incontinence procedure. The extent of the evaluation depends on the complexity of the presentation.

The degree of ISD should be assessed preoperatively using a combination of assessment tools. In the history, patients who have only hypermobility describe leakage with vigorous activity, whereas patients with ISD tend to have leakage with minimal activity. On physical examination, patients with incontinence due to hypermobility have descent of the urethra and bladder neck during stress maneuvers. On the other hand, reproducible demonstration of stress incontinence through a normally supported urethra is suggestive of ISD. Corroboration of ISD may be established by a variety of tests, including leak point pressure, passive urethral profilometry, imaging techniques such as fluoroscopy, and on occasion cystoscopic assessment. Most of these assessment tools do not provide a definitive diagnosis alone, especially if the patient has coexistent DI, which can cause a functional opening of the bladder neck at rest. Therefore, the entire clinical presentation must be considered.

Procedures for Hypermobility. After complete evaluation, if the primary pathophysiologic defect appears to be urethral hypermobility or displacement, three main types of procedures are used:

- Retropubic suspension.

- Needle bladder neck suspension.

- Anterior vaginal repair.

Retropubic or needle suspension is recommended for women with hypermobility when SUI is the primary indication for surgery. On the basis of greater efficacy, these procedures are recommended over anterior vaginal repair for hypermobility. (Strength of Evidence = B.)

Review of the available literature shows that in general retropubic and needle suspension procedures produce a superior result to that of anterior repair in "curing" UI. This analysis of results usually focuses exclusively on the symptom of stress incontinence and does not account for postoperative problems such as the new development of an enterocele or rectocele large enough to require surgery, persistent voiding difficulty, or DI. Therefore, although the reported cure rate for stress incontinence is high, the number of women with an entirely satisfactory outcome may not be. Treatment must be individualized for each patient as well as standard recommendations about which operation will be best. The option selected depends on the surgeon's training and expertise and on the presence of concurrent pathology that would require correction by a vaginal or abdominal approach.

For hypermobility with coexisting ISD the surgical procedure should stabilize the anatomic support and compress the urethra, which invariably means using one of the sling procedures (see Procedures for ISD below). The choice must be individualized for each patient. Women who have severely damaged urethras require special procedures such as urethral or bladder neck reconstruction, urethral substitution, continent vesicotomy, or urinary diversion.

Management must be individualized for women whose primary problem is prolapse of the pelvic organs but who have SUI or in whom temporary replacement of the prolapse during preoperative evaluation uncovers SUI. In these circumstances, a decision about the most appropriate anti-incontinence procedure to be combined with repair of the prolapse should account for the type of SUI present (hypermobility or ISD), the operation chosen to repair the prolapse (abdominal or vaginal), and additional morbidity from the continence operation weighed against the degree of incontinence. Preoperative urodynamic examination should be performed if this information is needed to choose the type of operation to be performed.

Retropubic suspension. Retropubic suspension procedures include several different techniques performed through a low abdominal incision (i.e., retropubic approach). All techniques have in common elevation of the lower urinary tract, particularly the urethrovesical junction, within the retropubic space. The procedures differ according to what structures are used to achieve the elevation. For the Marshall-Marchetti-Krantz procedure, the periurethral tissue is approximated to the symphysis pubis. For the Burch colposuspension, the vaginal wall lateral to the urethra and bladder neck is elevated toward Cooper's ligament. The paravaginal repair involves reapproximating the endopelvic fascia to the pelvic wall at the arcus tendineus.

To evaluate this category of procedures, 45 studies incorporating 3,882 patients were reviewed (Baker and Drutz, 1992; Beck, Thomas, and Maughan, 1968; Bergman, Ballard, and Koonings, 1989; Bergman, Koonings, and Ballard, 1989a,b,c; Brieger and Korda, 1992; Duncan, Nurse, and Mundy, 1992; Eriksen, Hagen, Eik-Nes, et al., 1990; Fall, Erlandson, and Pettersson, 1984; Ferriani, de Sa, de Moura, et al., 1990; Francis, Sand, Hamrang, et al., 1987; Goodno and Powers, 1992; Green, McGuire, and Lytton, 1986; Hilton and Stanton, 1983; Iosif, 1985; Jouppila, Kauppila, Ylikorkala, et al., 1977; Kiilholma, Makinen, Chancellor, et al., 1993; Kil, Hoekstra, van der Meijden, et al., 1991; Korda, Ferry, and Hunter, 1989; Kujansuu, 1983; Langer, Ron-El, Newman, et al., 1988; Langer, Ron-El, Bukovsky, et al., 1988; Lockhart, Maggiolo, and Politano, 1983; Lose, Jorgensen, and Johnsen, 1988; Milani, Scalambrino, Quadri, et al., 1985; Morgan, 1973; Nielsen and Lundvall, 1973; Park and Miller, 1988; Penttinen, Kaar, and Kauppila, 1989; Penttinen, Lindholm, Kaar, et al., 1989; Pow-Sang, Lockhart, Suarez, et al., 1986; Richardson, Ramahi, and Chalas, 1991; Richmond and Sutherst, 1989a; Sand, Bowen, Ostergard, et al., 1988; Shull and Baden, 1989; Spencer, O'Conor, and Schaeffer, 1987; Stanton, Williams, and Ritchie, 1976; Stanton and Cardozo, 1979; Steel, Cox, and Stanton, 1985; Thunedborg, Fischer-Rasmussen, and Jensen, 1990; Van Geelen, Theeuwas, Eskes, et al., 1988; Vordermark, Brannen, Wettlauffer, et al., 1979; Wheelahan, 1990). Total "cure" rates averaged 79 percent, and 84 percent were "cured" or improved.

Overall complication rates reported for retropubic operations average 18 percent (6–57 percent). In the recent literature, complications reported among the studies of retropubic urethral suspensions were sparse, being included in only 6 of 13 papers with insufficient information and consistency to allow accurate statistical reporting. Wound infections, urinary retention, *de novo* DI, and dyspareunia were all noted in the 3–15 percent range. The cause of postoperative symptomatic enterocele/rectocele with anterior traction on the anterior wall seems to be most prominent after the Burch operation, occurring in up to 12 percent of patients (Kiilholma, Makinen, Chancellor, et al., 1993). Recently, some of these retropubic procedures have been performed laparoscopically.

Needle bladder neck suspension. Another type of anatomic correction employs needle suspension of the bladder neck. Variations of this procedure are all performed through a vaginal approach, and most utilize small suprapubic skin incisions (Cobb and Ragde, 1978; Gittes and Laughlin, 1987; Pereyra, Lebherz, Growdon, et al., 1982; Stamey, 1980; Raz, 1981). Anchoring tissues adjacent to the urethra and bladder neck are held by suspending sutures.

Of the 3,015 patients studied in the reviewed research, most had the Stamey procedure; the others had the Pereyra-Raz procedure (Abbassian, 1989; Ashken, 1990; Benderev, 1992; Benson, Agosta, and McClellan, 1990; Bergman, Ballard, and Koonings, 1989; Bergman, Koonings, and Ballard, 1989a,c; Bhatia and Bergman, 1985a; Bosman, Vierhout, and Huikeshoven, 1993; Cobb and Ragde, 1978; Dijkman and Friese, 1984; Duncan, Nurse, and Mundy, 1992; Foster and O'Reilly, 1989; Ganabathi, Abrams, Mundy, et al., 1992; Gaum, Ricciotti, and Fair, 1984; Griffith-Jones and Abrams, 1990; Hilton, 1989; Huland and Bucher, 1984; Jones, Shah, and Worth, 1989; Juma, Little, and Raz, 1992; Kil, Hoekstra, et al., 1991; Kirby and Whiteway, 1989; Kursh, 1992; Kursh, Angell, and Resnick, 1991; Leach and Raz, 1984; Lopez Lopez, Valdivia Uria, and Uca Terran, 1992; Loughlin, Whitmore, et al., 1990; Mundy, 1983; Netto, Lemos, Palma, et al., 1988; Nitti, Bregg, et al., 1993; Parra and Shaker, 1990; Penttinen, Kaar, and Kauppila, 1989; Pereyra, Lebherz, Growdon, et al., 1982; Pope, Shaw, Coptcoat, et al., 1990; Pow-Sang, Lockhart, Suarez, et al., 1986; Ramon, Mekras, and Webster, 1990; Raz, Sussman, Erickson, et al., 1992; Richardson, Ramahi, and Chalas, 1991; Shah and Holder, 1989; Spencer, O'Conor, and Schaeffer, 1987; Stamey, 1980; Varner, 1990; Walker and Texter, 1992; Wujanto and O'Reilley, 1989). For the combined series, 74 percent were continent postoperatively and 84 percent were "cured" or improved; followup varied. Complications included UTI, urinary retention longer than 3 weeks' duration, obstructive symptoms, suture abscess, wound infection or vaginal granuloma, vesicocutaneous fistula, hematoma, sutures pulling out of the vaginal fascia, sepsis, new onset of symptomatic DI, and prolonged suprapubic pain and *de novo* pelvic floor defects.

Anterior vaginal repair. The anterior vaginal repair category of treatments includes several modifications of the original Kelly plication. All techniques include some degree of dissection of the anterior vaginal wall from the overlying bladder base and urethra, and plication of the pubocervical fascia. The extent of the dissection and the location and extent of the placating (elevating) sutures vary substantially among these techniques. Although the success of these operations as a group is somewhat lower than retropubic or needle suspensions, some specific techniques achieve excellent success on objective followup, indicating the need to discriminate the actual technical details of each of these different operations before making generalizations (Beck, McCormick, and Nordstrom, 1991).

Review of 11 studies incorporating 957 patients reveals an overall "cure" rate of 65 percent (range = 31–91 percent) and a "cure" or improvement rate of 74 percent (range = 31–98 percent); followup varied (Beck, McCormick, and Nordstrom, 1991; Beck, Thomas, and Maughan, 1968; Bergman, Ballard, and Koonings, 1989; Bergman, Koonings, and Ballard, 1989c; Jouppila, Kauppila, Ylikorkala, et al., 1977; Kujansuu, 1983; Lose, Jorgensen, and Johnsen, 1988; Park and Miller, 1988; Stanton, Hilton, Norton, et al., 1982; Thunedborg, Fischer-Raumussen, and Jansen, 1990; Van Geelen, Theeuwes, Eskes, et al., 1988). Complication rates were provided for only two studies; the average was 14 percent.

Procedures for Intrinsic Sphincter Deficiency. Procedures for management of ISD include

- Sling procedures.

- Periurethral bulking injections.

- Placement of an artificial sphincter.

Sling procedures are recommended for women who have ISD with coexisting hypermobility or as first-line treatment for ISD. (Strength of Evidence = B.)

Periurethral bulking injections are recommended as first-line treatment for women with ISD who do not have coexisting hypermobility. (Strength of Evidence = B.)

Artificial sphincter is recommended for ISD patients who are unable to perform intermittent catheterization and have severe SUI that is unresponsive to other surgical treatments. Because of the high complication rate, this treatment is rarely used as primary therapy. (Strength of Evidence = B.)

Sling procedures. The various sling procedures all involve placing a sling, made of either autologous or heterologous material, under the urethrovesical junction and anchoring it to retropubic or abdominal structures or both. The operation can be performed through an abdominal approach, a vaginal approach, or a combined abdominal and vaginal approach. Sling operations are often performed in women with complicated incontinence, many of whom have failed previous attempts at surgical correction. The success and complication rate should be viewed with this fact in mind.

Data from a series of 9 studies of 434 patients with fascial slings indicated that 89 percent were "cured," and 92 percent were "cured" or improved (Beck, McCormick, and Nordstrom, 1988; Deppe, Castro-Marin, Nachamie, et al., 1978; Low, 1969; McGuire and Lytton, 1978; McIndoe, Jones, and Grieve, 1987; Narik and Palmrich, 1962; Ogundipe and Rosenzweig, 1992; Richmond and Sutherst, 1989a; Ridley, 1966). Combined analysis of 298 patients from six studies that used a synthetic sling indicated that 78 percent were "cured," and 84 percent were "cured" or improved (Brieger and Korda,

1992; Bryans, 1979; Kersey, 1983; Korda, Peat, and Hunter, 1989).

Although the total complication rate given for the fascial sling series was higher than that for the synthetic sling series, the synthetic sling caused more severe complications, many of which were directly attributable to local effects of the sling (i.e., erosion, nonhealing of the vaginal wall, abscess, vesicovaginal fistula). Fascial slings are preferable to synthetic slings because of the lower rate of local complications.

Data from 32 patients treated with the vaginal wall sling showed that 81 percent were dry, 9 percent were improved, and 9 percent showed no improvement (Ogundpipe and Rosenzweig, 1992; Ridley, 1966). Complications included urinary retention and new onset of irritative voiding symptoms.

Periurethral bulking injections involve the injection of materials such as polytetrafluoroethylene (PTFE), collagen, or autologous fat under cystoscopic guidance into an incompetent periurethral area. Patients being considered for periurethral collagen injection require a skin test for sensitivity to the material. Injection of the material appears to be technically easier because the number of patients requiring anesthesia or sedation is less than that reported with PTFE. The longevity of PTFE versus collagen has not been studied. Urinary tract infection and transient urethral irritation are the most common side effects after periurethral collagen injection. The procedures for periurethral bulking injections are described below in the section on male incontinence caused by ISD. In women, these injections are easily performed under local anesthesia. Combined data from 15 studies of 528 women indicate that after followup for up to 2 years 49 percent of patients were "cured" (range = 8–100 percent), and 67 percent were either "cured" or improved (Beckingham, Wemyss-Holden, and Lawrence, 1992; Berg, 1973; Deane, English, Hehir, et al., 1985; Eckford and Abrams, 1991; Harrison, Brown, and O'Boyle, 1993; Kiilhoma and Makinen, 1991; Lewis, Lockhart, and Politano, 1984; Lotenfoe, O'Kelly, Helal, et al., 1993; McGuire and Appell, 1994; O'Connell, McGuire, Aboseif, et al., in press; Santarosa and Blaivas, 1994; Schulman, Simon, Wespes, et al., 1983; Smart, 1991; Stricker and Haylen, 1993; Vesey, Rivett, and O'Boyle, 1988). Complications included urgency, UTI, and urinary retention.

Although documentation of teflon migration to the lung persisted (Claes and Stroobants, 1989) adverse reactions to this material in other sites has not been found. Increasing experience with collagen has established its efficacy in the short term, but, as with Teflon injection, long-term results beyond 5 years are not available.

Artificial sphincter. Artificial sphincter placement, described below in the section on ISD in men, has been used for women with ISD. Combined data from 8 studies of 192 women with ISD treated with artificial sphincter placement indicated that 77 percent were dry, and 80 percent were "cured" or improved (Appell, 1988; Light and Scott, 1985; Diokno, Hollander, and Alderson, 1987; Duncan, Nurse, and Mundy, 1992; Karram, Rosenzweig, and Bhatia, 1993; Motley and Barrett, 1990; Parulkar and Barrett, 1990; Webster,

Perez, Khoury, et al., 1992). Complications included fluid leak, loose cuff, erosion or atrophy of the cuff site, tubing kink, and infection.

Stress Incontinence in Men: Intrinsic Sphincter Deficiency

An underactive outlet in men may result from a congenital defect or from direct or indirect trauma to the anatomy or physiology of the bladder outlet. Direct trauma due to prostatectomy is the most common cause of sphincter insufficiency. Neurologic dysfunction (e.g., sympathetic innervation to the bladder neck, pelvic nerve to the intrinsic sphincter, pudendal nerve to the external sphincter) may be a primary or contributory etiology. Devascularization or fibrosis, most commonly following radiation therapy or surgery, may also contribute to decreased closure pressure of the bladder outlet. The high incidence of mixed incontinence requires that an alteration in bladder function be considered and diagnosed before surgical intervention for decreased outlet resistance. Postprostatectomy incontinence is not always due to sphincter insufficiency but sometimes to detrusor dysfunction or both. Patients must be evaluated for other possible causes of incontinence, including obstruction, DI, and poor bladder compliance.

The choices for surgical treatment of male sphincter insufficiency include

- Periurethral bulking injections.

- Placement of an artificial sphincter.

The sling procedure has been used only occasionally in men, and the information available is insufficient for providing effective recommendations at this time.

The preoperative evaluation may require a cystoscopy, and a simple cystometry or complex videourodynamic studies, depending on the suspected etiology. Special care and followup are required in neurologically impaired individuals due to a significant incidence of bladder compliance changes following therapy to increase outlet resistance. Before injection or sphincter implantation, it is advisable to wait at least 6 months to a year and to have the patient undergo behavioral and pharmacologic intervention during the intervening months. If an artificial sphincter is being considered, it is important to assess whether the patient has enough manual dexterity and ability to operate the device.

Periurethral Bulking Injections

Periurethral bulking injections are recommended as a first-line surgical treatment for men with ISD. (Strength of Evidence = B.)

Periurethral bulking injections can improve urinary loss in men with stress incontinence. The mechanism for improvement after injection therapy is still unclear but may reflect an improvement in urethral coaptation and possibly compression. Periurethral injections are less likely to succeed in male than in female patients and in all patients who have undergone pelvic radiation therapy or who have extensive periurethral scarring. Success is more common in patients who have stress incontinence after transurethral or open prostatectomy than in those after radical prostatectomy. The literature does not support the use of bulking agents in men with severe postprostatectomy incontinence (Appell, 1994). Experience and followup are limited for treatment by injections with collagen and fat, which are absorbed by patients over time. There are no randomized studies comparing the efficacy of different materials or of injection therapy with other forms of treatment. The analysis included 9 studies of 1,005 men treated with periurethral injection (Kaufman, Lockhart, Silverstein, et al., 1984; Corrie, Rodriguez, and Thompson, 1989; Deane, English, Hehir, et al., 1985; McGuire and Appell, 1994; Osther and Rohl, 1988; Smart, 1991; Stanisic, Jennings, et al., 1991; Politano, 1992; Santarosa and Blavias, 1994). Sample sizes ranged from a minimum of 3 to a maximum of 720. The mean age was 69 years, and mean followup time was 2.0 years. The "cure" rate was reported in eight studies and ranged from 0 to 66 percent, with a mean of 20 percent. The "cure"–improvement rate was reported in nine studies and ranged from 0 to 81 percent, with a mean of 42 percent.

Complications reported with PTFE included infection, urinary retention, fever, temporary erectile dysfunction, periurethral inflammatory reaction, extrusion of the material into the urine or perineal area, and burning sensation or perineal discomfort. Particles of PTFE have been found in patients' lungs after periurethral injection of PTFE, but the exact incidence and the clinical significance of this migration are not known.

Placement of an Artificial Sphincter

Artificial sphincter may be elected for ISD during the 6 months after prostatectomy. Behavioral intervention should also be tried during this period. (Strength of Evidence = B.)

Before periurethral injection therapy became available, placement of an artificial urinary sphincter was the most commonly used surgical procedure for the treatment of underactive outlet in men. Data on the current rate of comparative utilization of these two techniques are not available. Before implantation, urodynamic evaluation to confirm a stable, compliant, low pressure bladder is critical.

The analysis included 10 studies that presented data on 346 men, with sample sizes ranging from 11 to 96 (Brito, Mulcahy, Mitchell, et al., 1993; Gundian, Barrett, and Parulkar, 1989; Marks and Light, 1989; Nordling, Holm-Bentzen, and Hald, 1986; Lowe, Schertz, and Parsons, 1988; Malloy, Wein, and Carpiniello VL, 1989; Motley and Barrett, 1990; Schreiter, 1985; Wang and Hadley, 1991; Warwick and Abrams, 1990). The average age of the patients was 61.4 years. The "cure" rate was presented in nine studies and ranged from 33 to 88 percent, with a mean of 66 percent. The "cure" or improvement rate in the 10 studies ranged from 75 to 94.5 percent, with a mean of 85.3 percent.

Initial preoperative complications are mainly associated with urethral or bladder injury during implantation. Delayed complications included mechanical problems such as pump malfunction, fluid leak, or tubing kink; infection; or cuff-related site atrophy, incomplete compression, or erosion. In addition, urethral injury, pump erosion, and herniated reservoir were reported in fewer patients.

The utilization of the artificial urinary sphincter in patients after radiation therapy, cryotherapy, or pelvic fracture with urethroplasty is controversial because of concern about compromising the urethral blood supply. Also controversial is the use of intermittent catheterization after sphincter implantation. The experience of the implanting surgeon may be related to the incidence of complications.

Urge Incontinence: Detrusor Instability

Use of surgical procedures in the management of urge incontinence is uncommon. Surgical treatment is usually considered only in highly symptomatic patients in whom nonoperative management has failed repeatedly.

The surgical procedures reviewed for the treatment of overactive bladder include

- Augmentation intestinocystoplasty or urinary diversion.

- Bladder denervation procedures.

Augmentation intestinocystoplasty is recommended for those patients with intractable, severe bladder instability or poor bladder compliance that is unresponsive to nonsurgical therapies. (Strength of Evidence = B.)

Urinary diversion is recommended in severe intractable cases of detrusor instability or poor bladder compliance that is unresponsive to other therapies. (Strength of Evidence = C.)

Augmentation Intestinocystoplasty or Urinary Diversion. Various surgical procedures have been proposed for treating intractable, severe bladder instability and poor compliance. Augmentation cystoplasty with a patch of detubularized intestine is usually considered the procedure of choice. Urinary diversion with a urostomy or continent urinary diversion may be utilized as a last resort.

The risks of augmentation cystoplasty, in addition to those of any bowel surgery, include voiding difficulties that may require catheterization, mucus or stone formation, metabolic decompensation, and the rare long-range possibility of tumor formation. Contraindications for augmentation cystoplasty include renal insufficiency, bowel disease, intractable urethral disease, and inability to perform self-catheterization.

Twelve articles were reviewed (Bramble, 1982; Fenn, Conn, German, et al., 1992; George and Russel, 1991; Kockelbergh, 1991; Linder, Leach, and Raz, 1983; Lockhart, Ellis, Helal, et al., 1990; Mundy and Stephenson, 1985; Raz, Ehrlich, Zeidman, et al., 1988; Robertson, Davies, et al., 1991; Sethia, Webb, and Neal, 1991; Sidi, Becher, Reddy, et al., 1990; Strawbridge, Kramer, Castillo, et al., 1989). The studies included 403 subjects, with sample sizes ranging from 11 to 112. The mean age was 35.8 years and the known mean followup was 2.2 years (four studies). All studies included both men and women but did not separate out results. Thirty-eight percent of patients were rendered continent with spontaneous voiding (range 0–87 percent). If patients continent with CICS are included, then the mean "cure" rate is 82 percent (range 56–100 percent) and the improvement rate is 90 percent (71–100 percent).

Complications included recurrent UTI (29 patients), persistent mucus formation (11 patients), hourglass stricture at the vesicocecal anastomosis (1 patient), and complications from the artificial sphincter (3 mechanical problems, 1 pump erosion, 1 cuff erosion). The total complication rates were 47 of 87 (54 percent) for the augmentation and 5 of 22 (44 percent) for the artificial sphincter.

Bladder Denervation Procedures. Subtrigonal phenol injections (Blackford, Murray, Stephenson, et al., 1984; Ewing, Bultitude, and Shuttleworth, 1982; Nordling, Steven, Meyhoff, et al., 1986; Rosenbaum, Shaw, and Worth, 1990; Wall and Stanton, 1989) and bladder denervation (Alloussi, Loew, Mast, et al., 1984; Diokno, Hollander, and Alderson, 1987; Hodgkinson and Drukker, 1977; Lucas, Thomas, Clarke, et al., 1988; McGuire and Savastano, 1984; Opsomer, Klarskov, Holm-Bentzen, et al., 1984; Rockswald, Chou, and Bradley, 1978; Torring, Petersen, Kelmar, et al., 1988) are not presently recommended because the "cure" rates are low, and therefore the risk-to-benefit ratio is too great.

Subtrigonal or transvesical phenol injection. Five series of patients treated with subtrigonal phenol injections were reviewed and combined to include a total of 244 patients (Blackford, Murray, Stephenson, et al., 1984; Ewing, Bultitude, and Shuttleworth, 1982; Nordling, Steven, Meyhoff, et al., 1986; Rosenbaum, Shaw, and Worth, 1990; Wall and Stanton, 1989). "Cure" was not defined in all studies, but a short-term ($\leq$ 6 months) response was reported in 142 patients. Almost all patients had relapsed by 2 years, however. For the combined series, complications included trigonal ulcer, vesicovaginal fistula, hematuria, vesicoureteral reflux, partial sciatic nerve palsy, obstructive voiding symptoms, and permanent urinary retention. The total complication rate was 12.3 percent.

Of these five studies subjected to meta-analysis, two reported treating both men and women (Nordling, Steven, Meyhoff, et al., 1986; Rosenbaum, Shaw, and Worth, 1990), and the other three included female patients only. Combined analysis of all male subjects revealed that the phenol injection produced no "cure" or improvement. Of the 234 female subjects, 8.6 percent were "cured" and an average of 52.5 percent were "cured" or improved.

Thus, transvesical phenol injection appears to be totally ineffective in "curing" or improving male continence, ineffective in "curing" female incontinence, and only possibly effective in improving female incontinence.

Bladder denervation. Eight studies of bladder denervation were reviewed. In three, bladder denervation was used to treat idiopathic DI in patients with no demonstrable neurologic lesions (Alloussi, Loew, Mast, et al., 1984; Diokno, Vinson, and McGillicuddy, 1977; Hodgkinson and Drukker, 1977). Three other studies examined patients with DH from known neurologic problems (McGuire and Savastano, 1984; Rockswald, Chou, and Bradley, 1978; Torring, Peterson, Kelmar, et al., 1988). Two studies included patients in both categories (Lucas, Thomas, Clarke, et al., 1988; Opsomer, Klarskov, Holm-Bentzen, et al., 1984).

The three studies concerning only idiopathic DI included a total of 52 patients (Alloussi, Lowe, Mast, et al., 1984; Diokno, Vinson, and McGillicuddy, 1977; Hodgkinson and Drukker, 1977). Denervation was accomplished by selective sacral rhizotomy, S3 foramen injection, or transvaginal denervation. Only 20 patients had a stated followup period longer than 1 year. Combined analysis of all treated patients revealed an average of 40.4 percent "cured" and an average of 59.4 percent "cured" or improved. The only complication listed was perineal hypoesthesia.

The three studies concerning only true neurologic disease included 34 patients (McGuire and Savastano, 1984; Rockswald, Chou, and Bradley, 1978; Torring, Peterson, Kelmar, et al., 1988). Twenty-three had multiple sclerosis, nine had paraplegia or quadriplegia, and two had cerebral lesions. Denervation was accomplished by selective sacral rhizotomy in 19, sacral rhizotomy in 12, and 2–4 dorsal root ganglionectomy in three. Followup ranged from 2 to 10 years. Combined analysis of all treated patients revealed an average of 47.1 percent "cured" or improved. Complications included one wound infection and two episodes of intra-operative bleeding. The two studies concerning both types of instability were the only studies in which long-term followup (at least 4 years) was reported for all patients after selective sacral rhizotomy (Opsomer, Klarskov, Holm-Bentzen, et al., 1984; Lucas, Thomas, Clarke, et al., 1988). Thirteen patients (50 percent) had either persistent or recurrent incontinence, and six others were dry only with additional treatment with anticholinergics. Thus, the long-term results were not favorable.

Overflow Incontinence: Bladder Neck or Urethral Obstruction

Symptoms of overflow or incontinence secondary to urethral obstruction can be addressed with a surgical procedure to relieve the obstruction. (Strength of Evidence = B.)

Intermittent catheterization or an indwelling catheter may be considered in patients who are not candidates for surgery and suffer overflow incontinence due to urethral obstruction. (Strength of Evidence = C.)

There is no evidence to support the use of urethral dilation for the treatment of incontinence in women, although it may be useful in the extremely rare cases of primary obstruction. (Strength of Evidence = C.)

Internal urethrotomy is not recommended for treating urethral obstruction in women. (Strength of Evidence = C.)

Overflow incontinence should be ruled out during the basic evaluation. PVR volume can be evaluated by catheterization or by pelvic ultrasound. If overflow incontinence is discovered, its cause—anatomic obstruction, detrusor weakness, or both—should be determined.

A patient with a persistently underactive detrusor with or without obstruction is best treated by intermittent catheterization (IC). A patient with an underactive detrusor and outlet obstruction has a significantly lower chance of favorable surgical outcome than a patient with normal detrusor activity. If the patient or caregivers are unable to perform urethral catheterization, other options include indwelling urethral or suprapubic drainage, or supravesical diversion.

If the etiology is anatomic obstruction with an adequately contracting detrusor and the patient has an acceptable level of surgical risk, the best treatment is surgery.

The Female Patient. In women, anatomic obstruction can result from prior anti-incontinence surgery or severe pelvic prolapse. For women who have anatomic obstruction after anti-incontinence surgery, two procedures can relieve the obstruction. Obstruction from an endoscopic needle bladder neck suspension can be relieved by cutting one of the suspending sutures. To evaluate the outcome of this procedure, five studies were reviewed (Araki, Takamoto, Hara, et al., 1990; Fowler, 1986; Huland and Bucher, 1984; Mundy, 1983; Vordermark, Brannen, Wettlauffer, et al., 1979). The combined series of 4 studies included 182 patients who had had a needle bladder neck suspension. Ten patients (5 percent) developed obstructive voiding symptoms, which were resolved after one suture was out; only one patient had a recurrence of incontinence.

The other procedure—urethrolysis (remobilization of the periurethral adhesions) with or without resuspension—can be used after almost any type of anti-incontinence surgery. Three studies included 41 patients who were classified by symptoms and urodynamic studies and underwent urethrolysis through a transvaginal approach in combination with a repeat endoscopic suspension regardless of the presence or absence of preoperative incontinence (McGuire, Letson, and Wang, 1989; Nitti and Raz, 1994; Zimmern, Hadley, Leach, et al., 1987). Seventy-one percent of the patients had improved voiding patterns by urodynamic evaluation, and 80 percent had some improvement in symptoms, with 79 percent of those who were incontinent preoperatively exhibiting resolution of their stress incontinence.

The Male Patient. In elderly men, the most common cause of anatomic obstruction is benign prostatic hyperplasia (BPH). The treatment of BPH is multifaceted and is addressed in *Benign Prostatic Hyperplasia: Diagnosis and Treatment. Clinical Practice Guideline.*

Other Measures and Supportive Devices

Other measures and supportive devices used in the management of UI include the following:

- Intermittent catheterization.

- Indwelling urethral catheterization.

- Suprapubic catheters.

- External collection systems.

- Penile compression devices.

- Pelvic organ support devices.

- Absorbent pads or garments.

Intermittent Catheterization

IC is recommended as a supportive measure for patients with spinal cord injury, persistent UI, or chronic urinary retention secondary to underactive or partially obstructed bladder. (Strength of Evidence = B.)

IC has become standard treatment for persons with spinal cord injuries and for patients with other forms of chronic urinary retention due to an underactive or partially obstructed bladder. This procedure can be performed by patients or their caregivers using sterile or clean catheters to provide intermittent routine bladder emptying every 3–6 hours. Long-term use of IC appears preferable to indwelling catheterization in regard to complications such as infections and bladder and renal stones; however, well-designed comparison studies have not been performed (Webb, Lawson, and Neal, 1990; Warren, 1990). In spinal cord patients, the incidence of bacteriuria is 1–3 percent per IC, and between one and four episodes per 100 days of catheterization using IC four times a day (Warren, 1994). Other complications include urethral inflammation, stricture, false passage, hydronephrosis, and epididymitis (Webb, Lawson, and Neal, 1990).

Clean technique for IC is recommended for young, male, neurologically impaired individuals. (Strength of Evidence = B.)

Sterile technique for IC is recommended for elderly patients and patients with compromised immune system. (Strength of Evidence = C.)

IC may be performed as a clean or sterile procedure among young, neurologically impaired individuals. The nonsterile clean approach appears to result in rates of infection lower than those noted with indwelling catheters. Furthermore, the infections that do occur are usually managed without complication provided vesicourethral reflux does not exist, and bladder overdistension and trauma are avoided (Diokno, Sonda, Hollander, et al.,

1983; Perkash and Giroux, 1993; Wyndaele and Maes, 1990).

King, Carlson, Mervine, et al. (1992) compared the incidence of urinary tract infection (UTI) using sterile and clean procedures in 46 randomly assigned, hospitalized, young patients with spinal cord injuries. Sterile catheter kits and procedures were utilized during IC of 23 subjects, and the remainder used the clean technique but did use a new sterile catheter every 24 hours. Results showed no statistical differences in symptomatic or asymptomatic infections between the two groups. The investigators recommended the use of a new sterile catheter every 24 hours if the clean procedure is used.

A followup study of clean IC in 50 nonhospitalized male patients with spinal cord injuries (mean age = 46; range = 19–70 years), with a followup period of 3 months–6.5 years (mean of 22 months), reported that 43 of the 50 subjects (86 percent) developed significant bacteriuria, and 31 genitourinary complications occurred in 21 patients (Perkash and Giroux, 1993). The investigators concluded that clean intermittent catheterization can be a long-term management approach for spinal cord patients; however, this intervention is not without risk of secondary complications. Thus, close monitoring is required so that early and effective treatment can be provided to prevent serious problems. Furthermore, the investigators also noted that maintenance of acceptable intravesical pressures with the use of anticholinergic therapy was important in avoiding serious complications in this group of patients.

The susceptibility of older persons to develop nosocomial infections puts them at higher risk than younger persons for developing bacteriuria and other complications caused by IC. Elderly and other persons with impaired immune systems and atrophic mucosa are also at risk (Terpenning, Allada, and Kauffman, 1989; Warren, 1990). Although the incidence of infection and other complications for elderly patients using sterile versus clean IC is not well established, it appears that sterile IC is the safest method for this high-risk population (Terpenning, Allada, and Kauffman, 1989). Older persons who have the physical and cognitive abilities and who are motivated can be taught to perform IC. A caregiver can also be instructed to perform IC for impaired individuals.

Routine use of long-term suppressive therapy with antibiotics in patients with chronic, clean IC is not recommended. (Strength of Evidence = B.)

In high-risk populations, for example, those with an internal prosthesis or those who are immunosuppressed because of age or disease, the use of antibiotic therapy for asymptomatic bacteriuria must be individually reviewed. (Strength of Evidence = C.)

As a general rule, the use of long-term suppressive therapy with antibiotics in people regularly using clean IC is undesirable because it is associated with the emergence of resistant bacterial strains. It is generally agreed that symptomatic UTI should be treated. In high-risk populations, for example, those with an internal prosthesis or those who are immunosuppressed because of age or disease, the use of antibiotic therapy for asymptomatic bacteriuria must be individually reviewed (Joseph, Jacobson, Strausbaugh, et al., 1991; Wahlquist, McGuire, Greene, et al., 1983). Controlled trials are needed to further evaluate the benefit–risk ratio of these methods of continence management.

Indwelling Urethral Catheters

Indwelling catheters may be recommended as a supportive measure for patients whose incontinence is caused by obstruction and for whom other interventions are not feasible. Indwelling catheters are recommended for selected incontinent patients who are terminally ill or for patients with pressure ulcers as short-term treatment. (Strength of Evidence = B.)

Indwelling catheters are recommended in severely impaired individuals in whom alternative interventions are not an option and when a patient lives alone and a caregiver is unavailable to provide other supportive measures. (Strength of Evidence = C.)

An indwelling urethral (Foley) catheter is a closed sterile system inserted through the urethra to allow bladder drainage. The use of indwelling catheters should be restricted to persons whose incontinence is caused by urinary tract obstruction that cannot otherwise be treated and for which alternative therapy is not feasible. Examples include acutely ill persons for whom incontinence interferes with necessary monitoring of fluid balance and terminally ill or severely impaired persons for whom bed and clothing changes are painful or disruptive. In situations where the severity of the incontinence and the complexity of the person's care have contributed to skin irritation or pressure ulcers (Stage III or IV), an indwelling catheter may be indicated for short-term therapy until the skin condition resolves.

Studies suggest that approximately 50 percent of nursing home patients are incontinent and that approximately 2–4 percent may require urinary catheterization; however, the actual prevalence of use of indwelling catheters measured in several nursing homes ranges from 6 to 28 percent (Ouslander, Kane, and Abrass, 1982; Warren, Steinberg, Hebel, et al., 1989). Indwelling catheter use in the homebound patient is common and requires supervision by a registered nurse and additional personal hygiene care by paraprofessionals. The use of these devices in homebound individuals increases the cost of caring for these persons.

Long-term use of indwelling catheters is a significant cause of bacteriuria and UTI. Bacteriuria, which may be caused by encrustation formation of mineral and bacteria complexes, develops in most persons within 2–4 weeks after catheter insertion (Bjork, Pelletier, and Tight, 1984; Cox, Hukins, and Sutton, 1989; Tenney and Warren, 1988; Warren, Muncie, and Hall-Craggs,

1988). Cases of sepsis and death from severe UTI have been reported. In a nursing home population, mortality was three times higher in those with indwelling catheters than in noncatheterized patients, with significantly increased mortality in catheterized females (Kunin, Chin, and Chambers, 1987a,b). Other complications associated with indwelling catheters include obstruction secondary to encrustation, leakage, unprescribed removal, pain, bladder spasms, urethral erosion, stones, epididymitis, urethritis, periurethral abscess, chronic renal inflammatory changes, fistula formation, hematuria, and urinary leakage (Kunin, 1989; Warren, Muncie, and Hall-Craggs, 1988). Patients who are being managed with indwelling catheters over a long period of time should have their bladders evaluated by urologists on a routine basis.

Management of indwelling catheters varies. The usual practice is to change indwelling catheters every 30 days, but no data are available on the optimal frequency of catheter changes. Patients found to have encrustations and blockage might do better if their catheters were changed more frequently than every 30 days (Kunin, Chin, and Chambers, 1987a). If the patient has symptomatic UTI, the entire catheter and system must be changed and a new urine culture obtained when the new catheter is inserted (Grahn, Norman, White, et al., 1985; Rubin, Berger, Zodda, et al., 1980). No studies have identified an ideal catheter size, balloon size, or type of indwelling catheter, although most experts agree that the standard catheter size is 14FR, 16FR, or 18FR with a 5-cc balloon filled with 10 cc of sterile water. There is evidence to refute the practice of catheter irrigation and clamping before removal; in addition, disinfection of urinary drainage bags is ineffective in preventing infection (Thompson, Haley, Searcy, et al., 1984). Routine bladder irrigation of catheters not only is ineffective in eradicating bacteriuria but also may further disrupt the already damaged bladder epithelium, predisposing the patient to further infection (Elliott, Gopal Rao, Reid, et al., 1987; Ruwaldt, 1983). Routine irrigation is not recommended if obstruction occurs. In patients with frequent obstruction, the system should be changed and other types of catheters or alternative management should be considered. A person with an indwelling catheter must be reassessed periodically to determine whether a voiding trial or bladder retraining program might be effective in eliminating the need for the catheter or whether surgical risk might now be improved such that a surgical procedure could be performed to relieve obstruction.

It is not known which type of catheter (e.g., silicone, latex, Teflon) is best. Specific risks are difficult to assess because studies generally do not report the type or brand of catheter used. The development of silver-coated, antimicrobial, lubricous-coated, and female catheters may decrease the formation of encrustation and other complications; however, further research on these products is needed to determine their effectiveness (Blacklock, 1986; Brocklehurst, Hickey, Davies, et al., 1988; Johnson, Roberts, Olsen, et al., 1990; Kunin and Finkelberg, 1971; Liedberg and Lundeberg, 1990; Liedberg, Lundeberg, and Ekman, 1990).

Suprapubic Catheters

Suprapubic catheters are for short-term use following gynecologic, urologic, and other surgery, or as an alternative to long-term catheter use. Suprapubic catheterization is contraindicated as a long-term management option in persons with chronic unstable bladder (DI, DH) and ISD. (Strength of Evidence = B.)

Suprapubic catheterization involves percutaneous or surgical introduction of a catheter into the bladder through the anterior abdominal wall. Indications include short-term use following gynecologic, urologic, and other types of surgery or as an alternative to long-term catheter use in men and in women with urethral closure. Suprapubic catheters are contraindicated in persons with chronic unstable bladder (DI, DH) or ISD. Stower, Massey, and Feneley (1989) treated 50 patients with diagnoses of neurogenic bladder with suprapubic catheterization and urethral closure. Patients in this series had either severe neurologic disease or pressure ulcers, or had refused an ileal conduit. Complications included leakage around the catheter (17 percent), bladder stone formation (21 percent), symptomatic UTI (90 percent), and recurrent blocked catheter (10 percent).

Barnes, Shaw, Timoney, et al. (1993) studied 40 outpatients (23 women, 17 men) with a mean age of 45 years in whom suprapubic catheters were used to manage UI over a 2-year period. Thirty-five of the subjects had suffered traumatic spinal cord injury, and five had spinal cord lesions of nontraumatic origin. All had failed or declined to use IC to empty their bladders. Catheter-related problems were common, and only five patients had experienced no problems since insertion. The researchers reported good results utilizing size 14–16 French catheters, anticholinergic drug therapy, and daily clamping of the catheter. Only patients not using the medication and daily clamping regimen experienced reflux and decrease in bladder capacity. Leakage from the urethra and blocking of the catheter was reported for five patients. No discussion of problems with bacteriuria was presented. Immediate complications included cellulitis, hematoma, and bowel injury of 32 patients who expressed an opinion; 27 were satisfied with this form of bladder management. Long-term complications were similar to those associated with the use of indwelling catheters (Feneley, 1983; Stower, Massey, and Feneley, 1989).

Further studies are needed on the use of suprapubic catheterization for long-term management of UI. In the absence of data, panel consensus is that a suprapubic catheter is preferable to an indwelling catheter in the patient who requires chronic bladder drainage and for whom no other alternative therapy is possible, because it eliminates urethral complications. However, management of suprapubic catheters presents potential problems such as uncontrolled urine leakage, skin erosion, and hematoma, and problems with catheter reinsertion. Long-term medical management of suprapubic catheterization may also be problematic if health care providers lack knowledge and expertise and if the homebound patient lacks quick access to medical care if a problem arises. Suprapubic catheterization may be preferable to urethral catheters; however, additional studies are needed to better describe the benefits and risks of this treatment.

External Collection Systems

External collection systems are recommended for incontinent men and women who have adequate bladder emptying, who have intact genital skin, and in whom other therapies have failed or are not appropriate. (Strength of Evidence = C.)

External (condom) systems for men are catheters or devices made from latex rubber, polyvinyl, or silicone that are secured on the shaft of the penis by a double-sided adhesive, latex inflatable cuff, jockey's type strap, or foam strap, and connected to urine collecting bags by a tube. Condom catheters should not be used in patients with chronic obstruction. Frail, elderly males with cognitive impairment, who are considered candidates for condom catheter use, should be evaluated for symptomatic UTI, urinary retention, and upper tract damage before using these devices.

Patients and their caregivers should be carefully instructed in the proper application of external catheters and taught to check for possible complications. Although external catheters are preferable to indwelling catheters, they are also associated with UTI (Johnson, 1983; Ouslander, Greengold, and Chen, 1987b). Mechanical irritation and penile constriction may also occur from the friction caused by an external catheter (Jayachandran, Mooppan, and Kim, 1985). Therefore, the penis should be inspected daily, and careful attention must be given to avoid contact dermatitis, maceration of the penis, ischemia, and penile obstruction. Most complications result from improper and prolonged use of these devices. Also, persons with sensory loss secondary to neuropathy are unable to appreciate the potential for trauma to the area associated with improper use of the condom device (Jayachandran, Mooppan, and Kim, 1985).

Female external urine-collecting systems are available, but little research on their use and efficacy is available. External urine-collecting devices for women differ in their use of a vaginal locator, adhesive, suction, support belt, potential length of wear, and mobility with use (Pieper, Cleland, Johnson, et al., 1989). Johnson, O'Reilly, and Warren (1989) studied 63 applications of an external urine-collection device on incontinent women in a nursing home. The device was a flexible, plastic pouch that funneled urine through a connecting tube into a bedside collector. This device was allowed to remain *in situ* for a maximum of 48 hours. Only 14 percent of the devices required premature replacement because of unacceptable leakage. The primary adverse reaction was mild erythema. However, removal of the device was required for two patients with severe irritation and one patient with periurethral edema.

Johnson, Muncie, O'Reilly, et al. (1990) studied the use of external collecting devices in 26 women (mean age 79.8) residing in a rehabilitation center. Of 2,461 external device applications, almost 80 percent were adherent and leak free at 24 hours, and almost half were still adherent and leak free at 48 hours. There was no difference in mean wear time among 13 patients who were strictly bedridden; however, device leakage increased when a transfer (bed to chair) took place compared with no transfer. Periurethral erythema was observed in 1.6 percent of patients after removal of the device. The incidence of episodes of bacteriuria was 3.1 episodes per 100 days of external device use. Reported adverse reactions to the use of these devices include periurethral erythema and perineal itching (Johnson, Muncie, O'Reilly, et al., 1990; Johnson, O'Reilly, and Warren, 1989).

Penile Compression Devices

Penile compression devices are known to be used in clinical practice in the treatment of UI. No scientific literature was found to support the use of these devices. The panel recognizes the temporary use of penile compression devices in males in selected circumstances under the supervision of a health care provider. (Strength of Evidence = C.)

Mechanical devices for males, such as penile clamps, are reserved for temporary use in patients with ISD. Clamps must be removed at 3-hour intervals to empty the bladder. Several types are available; however, complications such as penile and urethral erosion, penile edema, pain, and obstruction can occur if clamps are improperly used.

Pelvic Organ Support Devices

Pessaries are recommended for women who have symptomatic pelvic organ prolapse. (Strength of Evidence = C.)

Data are not available to recommend or discourage the use of pessaries for the treatment of UI in women. (Strength of Evidence = C.)

Pessaries are devices made of rubber or silicone materials, or both, designed to reduce pelvic prolapse temporarily and alleviate symptoms of pelvic organ prolapse in females with and without incontinence. Pessaries are available in various sizes and shapes depending on the type and severity of prolapse and the integrity of the perivaginal muscles. Pessaries are recommended for women with symptomatic pelvic organ prolapse in two circumstances: (1) as a temporary measure for women awaiting surgical correction and (2) for treatment of women who are either unable, for medical reasons, or are unwilling to undergo correction of the prolapse. Use of the Smith Hodge vaginal pessary is reported to be an effective preoperative device for predicting the relative success of incontinence surgery for SUI (Bhatia and Bergman, 1985b). Objective evidence regarding their effectiveness in reducing UI has not been reported. Use of pessaries requires fitting and frequent and regular monitoring by trained health care providers. Complications can result when the pessary is misused or neglected and can include ulceration of the vagina and rectovaginal and vesicovaginal fistula (Goldstein, Wise, and Tancer, 1990). These devices should not be used in women with vaginal prolapse, in those who have vaginitis, or in those who cannot remove or insert the device without routine access to a health care provider.

A new vaginal device specifically designed to support the bladder neck in women with stress incontinence may hold promise for those who have sufficient manual dexterity and can learn to insert and remove the device. Davila and Osterman (1994) reported that of 30 physically active women studied, 25 were dry with the device. The mean number of weekly incontinent episodes decreased from 10 per week before treatment to 3 per week with the device in place ($P = 0.009$).

Absorbent Products

Absorbent products are recommended during evaluation, as an adjunct to other therapy, and for long-term care of patients with chronic, intractable urinary incontinence. (Strength of Evidence = C.)

Absorbent products and garments include the following:

- Shields, which are small absorbent perineal inserts.

- Guards, close-fitting products designed for light incontinence.

- Undergarments, which consist of full-length pads usually held in place by waist straps.

- Combination pad–pant systems.

- Adult diaper garments.

- Bed pads.

Absorbent pads and garments, either disposable or reusable, are widely used by persons with UI. Many community-dwelling persons use these products because of the protection they provide and because they can avoid seeking professional help for their problem. Others resort to pads because they have been dismissed rather than treated when seeking help for UI. From their perspective, absorbent products are a useful and rational way to manage the problem.

The widespread use of these products is reflected in the growth of the market of disposable pads and adult diapers from $99 million in 1972, to $173 million in 1982, to $496 million in 1987. Costs vary depending on the product and can be excessive for those on limited incomes. In 1987, these costs contributed to approximately half of the direct care costs for incontinence among residents in nursing homes (Sowell, Schnelle, Hu, et al., 1987). Although the quality and materials used in these products vary widely, little objective evaluation of disposable products has been conducted. Studies comparing cloth protective garments with disposable products have been conducted (Hu, Kaltreider, and Igou, 1990), but research comparing effectiveness and adverse effects of the various disposable products is lacking. Absorbent products are helpful during assessment and treatment of urinary incontinence. They also have a place as an adjunct to behavioral and other therapies, and in the care of persons with intractable incontinence. However, these products should not be used in place of therapeutic interventions to decrease or eliminate UI. Early dependency on absorbent pads may be a deterrent to continence, giving the wearer a sense of security and acceptance of the condition that removes the motivation to seek evaluation and treatment (Starer and Lobow, 1985). In addition, improper use of absorbent products may contribute to skin breakdown and UTI. Thus, appropriate use, meticulous care, and frequent garment changes are needed.

The following factors should be considered when absorbent products are used:

- Functional disability of the patient.

- Type and severity of incontinence.

- Gender.

- Availability of caregivers.

- Failure with previous treatment programs.

- Patient preference.

- Optimal product for individual patient.

- Skin integrity.

- Comorbidity.

- Incidence of vaginitis and bacteriuria.

- Quality of the product.

- Cost of the product.

In addition, it is recommended that the absorbent product industry standardize terminology and describe content and product performance (e.g., absorbency) to facilitate patient selection (National Kidney and Urologic Diseases Advisory Board, 1994). Research needs to be conducted to compare various factors of available products. Such studies would help health care providers make recommendations based on fact and will ultimately lead to the development of better products.

4 Chronic Intractable Urinary Incontinence

Prevalence and Incidence

The 1979 National Nursing Home Survey estimated the prevalence of UI in nursing homes at 50 percent (National Center for Health Statistics, 1979). A more recent study of 434 nursing home admissions reported the prevalence of incontinence to be 39 percent 2 weeks after admission (Palmer, German, and Ouslander, 1991). The incidence of new cases of incontinence after 1 year for the studied cohort was 27 percent, and remission during the same time period was 30 percent for women and 11 percent for men. The risk factors for UI included physical and mental impairment at both time periods.

Preliminary data from a survey of 8,400 home and hospice health agencies indicate that genitourinary conditions were among the 20 leading first-listed diagnoses for patients added to their caseloads (Strahan, 1994). An earlier study ascertained that UI was one of the 10 leading diagnoses for homebound individuals and first in total charges to Medicare for nursing services per person served (Ruther and Helbing, 1988). In a study of four home care programs in southern Ontario, an average of 22 percent of residents were assessed as incontinent (Mohide, Pringle, Robertson, et al., 1988). In a study of low-income, elderly individuals receiving publicly funded home care services, 23 percent were incontinent of urine and generated greater costs because of paraprofessional and other supportive care (Baker and Bice, 1995). In a study of family caregivers, 53 percent of care recipients were found to be incontinent (Noelker, 1987).

These data indicate that UI is common among both nursing home and home care populations. In addition, the number of disabled, dependent nursing home residents increased between 1977 and 1985 (Special Committee on Aging, 1988). Homebound individuals, by definition, either cannot leave their homes or do so with considerable difficulty as a result of a temporary or chronic disability (Strahan, 1994). The combination of decreased functional ability and UI is a particular challenge to caregivers in both settings. The magnitude of the problem of caring for incontinent homebound individuals will no doubt increase as the absolute number of aged persons increases and as maintenance of dependent, elderly persons at home becomes more common.

Assessment

Since 1990, nursing homes have been required by statute to perform standardized comprehensive assessment and screening of residents upon admission, annually, and when there is a significant change in condition. The Resident Assessment Instrument (RAI), which includes the Minimum Data Set (MDS) and utilization guidelines—including the Resident Assessment Protocols (RAPs) and triggers—was developed by the Health Care Financing Administration (HCFA) to improve the quality of care through maintenance and restoration of function (Health Care Financing Administration, 1995). When a patient is incontinent or has an indwelling catheter, assessment is performed using the UI RAP (Boulter, 1993; Resnick and Baumann, 1990). The RAP guides nurses and physicians through the evaluation process to ascertain the cause (including any reversible factors), chronicity (acute vs. chronic), and type of UI experienced by the patient (Resnick and Baumann, 1990). A stress test and evaluation of PVR volume are recommended, and general guidelines are provided for referral for additional evaluation.

The UI RAP does not include evaluation of daily voiding habits, or the frequency, volume, and circumstances of urinary incontinent episodes. Thus, an evaluation using bladder records should be added because it is often important to determine the frequency and severity of the UI to provide appropriate treatment (Wyman, Choi, Harkins, et al., 1988). Formalized assessment of cognitive function is a part of the RAPs. Instruments such as the Folstein Mini Mental State Examination (MMSE) may be helpful in selecting appropriate behavioral intervention (Folstein, Folstein, and McHugh, 1975). Recent data suggest that a short trial is pivotal to assessing responsiveness to a particular intervention (Ouslander, Schnelle, Uman, et al., 1995).

Fonda's (1990) definitions of continence status among short-term elderly rehabilitation patients and long-term nursing home residents in Australia can be helpful in evaluating and classifying incontinence. Fonda describes persons who have "independent continence" as those who are able to maintain continence without assistance. "Dependent continence" applies to persons who are physically or mentally impaired and are kept dry through the efforts of others. "Social continence" applies to those incapable of maintaining continence independently or through regular toileting by caregivers and who depend on absorbent products and other measures to contain urine leakage.

The combination of the RAP to assess incontinence and the use of Fonda's definitions can help in evaluating residents and selecting appropriate intervention. The MDS, RAP, and other evaluation tools, however, are not mandated for home care agencies providing skilled nursing visits. Thus, identification of hidden UI depends on the quality of continence questions included in each agency's nursing assessment, and on the skill and knowledge of the nurse. Research in the area of assessment and management of UI among homebound individuals has been performed by nurse investigators (McDowell, Engberg, Weber, et al., 1994; Rose, Baigis-Smith, Smith, et al., 1990). The negative psychological, physical, social, and financial impact of UI on homebound individuals and their caregivers points to the need for a systematic, consistent approach to this problem.

Interventions for Chronic UI

Care of persons with chronic UI should include attention to toileting schedules, fluid and dietary intake, strategies to decrease urine loss at

night, use of the most absorbent and skin-friendly protective garments possible, and prevention and early treatment of skin breakdown. (Strength of Evidence = B.)

Before a patient is classified as suffering from chronic intractable UI, the most appropriate intervention should be attempted. This guideline and the consensus of most experts suggest that if the person has stress, urge, or mixed UI, low-risk behavioral treatments should be attempted first if there are no contraindications. Persons with overflow UI who do not have a correctable obstruction may benefit from intermittent catheterization. Some patients may be candidates for surgical or pharmacologic interventions. However, side effects and complications of these treatments are major factors to consider in the treatment of dependent homebound or long-term care patients.

Behavioral Interventions

Studies indicate that behavioral interventions are effective if used by clinicians with training and experience in these methods. Success depends, in part, on using the most appropriate behavioral intervention for each patient. A method for correctly targeting behavioral interventions is to assess cognitive function using a formal test such as the Folstein MMSE (Folstein, Folstein, and McHugh, 1975). Persons who score within the normal range may benefit from interventions that require learning and recall abilities such as PME programs and bladder retraining (Burgio and Engel, 1990; Burns, Pranikoff, Nochajski, et al., 1990; Fantl, Wyman, McClish, et al., 1991; McDowell, Burgio, Dombrowski, et al., 1992; Wells, Brink, Diokno, et al., 1991). On the other hand, persons who demonstrate cognitive impairment on formal testing may benefit from scheduled voiding programs (e.g., prompted voiding or regular scheduled toileting) described in the Behavioral Techniques section of Chapter 3 of this guideline (Colling, Ouslander, Hadley, et al., 1992; Jirovec, 1991; Lekan-Rutledge, Hogue, and Miller 1992; Palmer, Bennett, Marks, et al., 1994; Schnelle, Newman, and Fogarty, 1990).

Toileting Assistance. Prompted voiding and regularly scheduled toileting are effective for preventing urinary accidents in some long-term care or homebound persons (Burgio, Engel, McCormick, et al., 1988; Schnelle, Newman, and Fogarty, 1990; Schnelle, Newman, Fogarty, et al., 1991). These toileting procedures require the assistance of staff, following a predetermined protocol. Prompted voiding programs require the discernment of wet or dry status and the ability to request toileting, whereas neither of these criteria is necessary for regularly scheduled toileting programs.

Several multisite clinical trials have studied a prompted voiding or scheduled toileting intervention strategy to decrease UI in nursing homes. One study using a 2-week baseline assessment and a 5-week intervention phase examined the effects of a prompted voiding intervention in 30 women whose average age was 85 (Creason, Grybowski, Burgener, et al., 1989). Objective evaluation using the Folstein MMSE and the Katz Activities of Daily Living (ADL) measure indicated that 65 percent had severe mental impairment and 78 percent had severe physical impairment. During the intervention, staff approached subjects hourly during waking hours and prompted them to void. Results showed that the experimental group's UI (i.e., percentage of time the patient was wet when checked) was reduced from 40 to 30 percent by the end of the study. The control group's UI increased from slightly more than four episodes to over five per day. Furthermore, all but one of those in the experimental group demonstrated definite patterns of UI that were incorporated into nursing care plans for toileting, and these patients showed continued improvement in UI status. Variations in staff adherence to the intervention may decrease the magnitude of the effect of this treatment.

In a 13-week behavioral therapy program in seven nursing homes carried out by project-trained research assistants 14 hours per day 7 days per week, 133 elderly women were checked hourly and prompted to toilet (Hu, Igou, Kaltreider, et al., 1989). Subjects' age averaged 85 years, and most were highly physically and mentally impaired as determined by the Katz ADL instrument and Folstein's MMSE. Subjects in the treatment group decreased the number of their wet episodes from 2 to 1.4 per day. Those who had severe incontinence, more physical dependence, and less mental impairment, as well as normal CMG and bladder capacity, responded better to the training program.

Schnelle, Newman, and Fogarty (1990) enrolled 126 subjects in a multiphase prompted treatment program. Subjects' average age was 82, the majority had severe mental impairment as determined on Folstein's MMSE, and only 11 percent could ambulate independently. During phase 1, which served as baseline, research staff checked each subject hourly for 12 hours per day over a 5-day period and changed them when they were wet. During phase 2, subjects were randomly assigned to immediate- and delayed-treatment groups for 5 days. Those in the immediate-treatment group were prompted to void every hour, asked if they were wet or dry, and then apprised of the accuracy of their response. Finally, they were asked to try to toilet, but were not toileted unless they requested assistance. Subjects were praised both for staying dry and for toileting successfully. Subjects in the delayed-treatment group continued to be checked hourly. Both the immediate and delayed groups participated in the prompted toileting treatment in phase 3. Subjects responded to prompted voiding as follows: 42 percent had less than one incontinent episode per 12 hours; 35 percent decreased their UI by two episodes per 12 hours but were still incontinent one or more times over the 12-hour period; and the rest did not reduce their UI by two or more episodes per 12 hours. The most successful subjects were less than 50-percent incontinent, could recognize when they needed to void, and had higher voided volumes and lower frequency of voiding.

Colling, Ouslander, Hadley, et al. (1992) conducted a clinical trial study among 88 subjects in four nursing homes over a 37-week period. Only subjects with urge or mixed UI were included in the study. Subjects' average age was 85, and all subjects were moderately to severely impaired, physically and mentally, as measured by the Katz ADL and the Short Portable Mental Status Questionnaire (SPMSQ). The study design consisted of a 12-week baseline period, a week during which subjects' individual patterns of voiding were established using an ambulatory electronic monitoring device over a 72-hour period, and a 12-week treatment period with habit training intervention carried out 24 hours per day 7 days per week, followed by a 12-week maintenance period. Data were gathered by research staff for one 24-hour period every 3 weeks throughout the duration of the study by checking subjects every hour. The intervention had three parts: nursing staff received a 4-hour inservice on how to accomplish the treatment, an individual toileting schedule was constructed for each subject based on the electronic monitoring data, and staff and patients received positive reinforcement for adhering to the toileting program and for successful toileting behavior, respectively (Harke and Richgels, 1992). Overall, the intervention significantly decreased UI for 86 percent of the experimental group, with one-third of the group improving more than 20 percent. Incontinence decreased an average of one episode per 24 hours for the entire group. Subjects with greater bladder capacity and less mental impairment responded best to treatment. There was resistance to changing nursing staff routines because of staff shortages, and nursing staff complied with the treatment regimen only 70 percent of the time.

Schnelle, Newman, Fogarty, et al. (1991) noted that 35 percent of nursing home residents were poor candidates for prompted voiding, specifically those who had frequent incontinent episodes, did not respond to prompts, and could not cooperate with toileting. Up to 40 percent of those in the study responded well. Responders can be identified by assessing their responsiveness to a 3-day trial of prompted voiding (Ouslander, Schnelle, Uman, et al., 1995). This may be true for homebound patients as well. Toileting persons according to their individual voiding habits (Colling, Ouslander, Hadley, et al., 1992) is an excellent means of avoiding accidents. If staff is untrained or undersupervised in nursing homes, this intervention is difficult; however, it provides caregivers of homebound patients with a viable management option.

Although research indicates that toileting interventions are promising, they may be compromised, depending on compliance of nursing staff (Campbell, Knight, Benson, et al., 1991; Schnelle, 1990). Nursing staff often expect total continence when these procedures are implemented and become disappointed when this does not occur (Schnelle, Newman, and Fogarty, 1990; Colling, Ouslander, Hadley, et al., 1992; Harke and Richgels, 1992). Several studies point to the importance of monitoring staff implementation of these procedures and providing feedback regarding performance (Burgio and Burgio, 1990; Schnelle, 1990). More research is needed to determine if using predictability of the resident's need to void for an individualized or fixed toileting schedule is more cost-efficient. Future studies should address formal mechanisms of performance appraisal and incentives to increase and maintain staff behaviors that affect patient outcomes. All studies, however, report a modest saving to institutions in laundry and supply costs with the decrease in incontinent episodes.

Homebound Patients. Although management of UI for homebound populations has not been as thoroughly studied as that for those receiving care in a nursing home or ambulatory care setting, two reports focused on the use of PME programs in homebound individuals. Rose, Baigis-Smith, Smith, et al. (1990) reported the successful use of PME training augmented by biofeedback therapy for cognitively intact home care subjects. McDowell, Engberg, Weber, et al. (1994) reported two case studies of severely disabled but cognitively intact homebound individuals who were successfully treated with a biofeedback-assisted PME program. A study of homebound elderly women found that women with UI had significantly less social interaction than continent women (Breakwell and Walker, 1988). Several studies are ongoing using a variety of treatment modalities for both cognitively impaired and cognitively intact homebound persons living in both urban and rural areas.

Physical and Environmental Alterations

All caregivers for elderly or disabled individuals must assess the environment in which the patient resides. Simple alterations, or the addition of toileting or ambulation devices, can often eliminate or reduce episodes of involuntary urine loss. (Strength of Evidence = C.)

Strategies that maintain or improve mobility are likely to prevent or reduce incontinent episodes in the frail elderly. (Strength of Evidence = B.)

Improvement of environmental factors such as access to toilets is likely to enhance treatment and may prevent UI in some cases. Persons who are cognitively intact but who have mobility or balance problems may be unable to suppress an urge until a caregiver arrives to toilet them, or, if they are independent, they are unable to walk or propel their wheelchair to the toilet in a timely fashion. These individuals may benefit from commodes or other external collecting devices such as urinals so that toileting can be achieved more easily. Other persons who can reach the bathroom may find the toilet inaccessible if grab bars and raised toilet seats are not in place.

Studies indicate that improved mobility is associated with remission of incontinence (Jirovec, 1991; Jirovec and Wells, 1990; Palmer, German, and Ouslander, 1991). These studies describe secondary prevention strategies and suggest that a simple walking exercise program not only increases mobility but also decreases the occurrence of UI.

Equipment that enhances mobility such as canes, walkers, and wheelchairs should be available for persons who have problems with ambulation. Toilets need to be at least 17 inches high with arms to assist the patient in lowering to or rising from the toilet seat. Some persons may be unable to reach the bathroom because of distance barriers such as furniture or other objects, poor lighting, or the need to climb stairs (McDowell, Engberg, Weber, et al., 1994). Chairs designed for ease in rising are especially helpful. In one study of elderly, institutionalized residents who were considered chairbound, 77 percent could rise unaided from a chair that was 17 inches at seat height and had arms 10 inches above the seat (Finlay, Bayles, Rosen, et al., 1983).

The use of restraints has been targeted as contributing to UI (Evans and Strumpf, 1990). Physical restraints include various straps and ties as well as "geri-chairs." In addition, sedating drugs can act as chemical restraints that also increase the potential for UI. It is now recognized that alternatives to restraints that maximize freedom of movement but ensure safety of the individual are almost always available.

Studies of specific environmental factors in the management of UI are inadequate to date. Those factors that discourage continence and promote incontinence should be identified and targeted for future research.

Fluid and Dietary Management

Constipation is a common problem for patients with chronic UI. Establishing a bowel regimen based on adequate fiber and fluid intake is often helpful. Elimination of bowel impaction and consequent pressure on the bladder and urethra are often necessary first steps in the treatment of chronic UI. (Strength of Evidence = C.)

Eliminating dietary caffeine such as in coffee, tea, colas, and chocolate is particularly important for persons with urge UI and frequency of urination (Crieghton and Stanton, 1990). However, limiting overall fluid intake is not effective for managing UI. Contrary to popular belief, maintaining adequate fluid intake is important especially for older adults who already have a decrease in total body water and are at risk for dehydration (Davis and Minaker, 1994; Schrier, 1990). In addition, inadequate fluid intake contributes to constipation. Routine use of stool softeners or laxatives should not be encouraged for management of bowel function and prevention of constipation. Laxatives are appropriate for facilitating bowel action prior to other management techniques including dietary fluids and physical activity, but should not be routinely used. Their use may be excessive and inappropriate in older adults. Emphasis should be on dietary measures such as high-fiber foods and fiber supplementation with unprocessed wheat bran and other high-fiber preparations, or the use of bulk-forming agents if dietary measures are neither feasible nor effective.

Management of Nocturia

Night-time voiding and incontinence are major problems for adults of all ages. Preventive measures to decrease night-time voids are recommended. The use of simple electronic urine detection devices should be encouraged for more efficient and effective patient monitoring of night-time urine loss. (Strength of Evidence = B.)

Persons who have nocturia greater than twice a night or who experience enuresis may benefit from fluid restriction and elimination of caffeine-containing beverages in the evening. These individuals should maintain adequate fluid intake by drinking the bulk of their liquids before dinner. Individuals who develop edema of the lower extremities during the day should be advised to elevate their lower extremities several hours during the late afternoon or evening to stimulate a natural diuresis and limit the amount of edema present at bedtime (O'Donnell, Beck, and Walls, 1990). In addition, the use of diuretics has been associated with lower night-time urine volumes; altering the timing of the administration of diuretics may decrease nocturia (Ouslander, Schnelle, Simmons, et al., 1993).

In a 10-day study of incontinence in 66 elderly, inpatient men, O'Donnell, Beck, and Walls (1990) found that the highest frequency of incontinent episodes occurred during the 4 p.m.–midnight shift, and the largest volume of urine loss per episode occurred during the night between midnight and 8 a.m. This study utilized an electronic sensor device to measure the frequency and used-pad weight to measure the volume of incontinent episodes. The lower level of physical activity and the mobilization of interstitial fluid that occurs in the supine position were cited as possible causes for these findings. A study by Ouslander, Schnelle, Simmons, et al. (1993), which measured the frequency and volume of urinary accidents for 136 male and female nursing home residents, showed that about 25 percent of the subjects produced significantly more urine at night than during the day.

Although larger studies are needed to better describe the time of day when urine production and excretion occurs, the findings of these two studies point to the need to reconsider continence care during the evening and night-time hours. The issues surrounding continence care during these times are complex and will require coordination of the efforts of long-term care managers, nurses, physicians, manufacturers, and researchers. Some of the issues include adequate staffing during evening and night-time hours, alterations in change routines, use of external collecting devices during these hours for both men and women, and the use of daytime diuretic therapy, as well as other measures described above to decrease edema and the volume of night-time urine production. The continued improvement of absorbent products and the correct use of skin cleaners, barrier creams, and powders are also important. Electronic urine detection devices may in some settings be useful to alert nursing staff of a patient's incontinent void. This would allow wet patients to be changed and permit dry patients to sleep uninterrupted by routine pad checks (O'Donnell, Beck, and Walls, 1990).

Other Measures and Supportive Care

Largely because of the introduction and emergence of behavioral therapies to treat UI during the past decade, the aim of continence experts and those who care for incontinent individuals has been to greatly decrease the indiscriminate use of such measures as absorbent pads and garments, external collecting devices, indwelling catheterization, and suprapubic catheters through the successful treatment of UI. However, these measures are beneficial for persons who fail treatment and remain incontinent, who are too ill or disabled to participate in behavioral programs, who cannot be helped by medications, or who have a type of UI that cannot be alleviated by surgical interventions. The judicious use of products to contain urine loss and maintain skin integrity are a first-line defense in these cases.

Protective garments and external collecting devices have a major part in the management of chronic incontinence. The most absorbent and skin-friendly products should always be utilized. However, no scientific literature is available to guide selection of the most effective product. (Strength of Evidence = C.)

Protective Pads and Garments. Absorbent products, classified as disposable or washable, include underpads, pant liners (shields and guards), adult diapers (briefs), and a variety of washable pants and disposable pad systems or combinations (Brink, 1990). In a survey questionnaire mailed to 36,500 Help for Incontinent People (HIP) members throughout the United States, more than 50 percent of the 10,427 respondents reported that they had used some form of protective garment (Jeter and Wagner, 1990). In addition, a survey of 512 community-dwelling elderly men and women with UI showed that 47 percent used absorbent products (Herzog, Fultz, Normalle, et al., 1989). Although there are no studies describing the prevalence of the use of protective garments among incontinent nursing home residents, results of most scheduled voiding programs in nursing homes directly indicate that disposable diapers or reusable pad and pant systems are used by their study subjects (Colling, Ouslander, Hadley, et al., 1992; Schnelle, Newman, Fogarty, et al., 1991).

Very little research has focused on these products despite their frequent use. Brink (1990, 1994) reported that of 30 studies performed between 1965 and 1987 and 14 studies between 1988 and 1993, all but 3 of the latter were performed outside of the United States. One study reported that continence care was labor intensive, requiring 25 minutes per day to change residents (Cella, 1988). In a cost study of UI in nursing homes, Hu, Kaltreider, and Igou (1990) randomly assigned 42 matched pairs of residents to treatment with either disposable or reusable cloth diapers. The total number of pads per day was 5.9 for the disposable pad users and 6.6 for those in the reusable pad treatment group. The average cost per day per person was $2.48 for disposable products and $2.61 for cloth products. Daily cost of disposable products when related to laundry cost revealed a lower daily cost for disposable products ranging from $0.44 to $0.68 or annual savings of $161–$248 per person. In addition, the skin of those using disposable products showed improvement after 1½ months; the skin of subjects using cloth pads and diapers deteriorated.

At present, there are no studies regarding the advantages or disadvantages of the various products available on the market. Data also are lacking comparing reusable with disposable products. Most evaluations are carried out by product manufacturers rather than independent researchers in the health care field and thus carry a bias. This limits their usefulness in assisting nurses, long-term care administrators, and consumers in deciding what products to use. Until objective information is available regarding patient comfort, ease of application and removal, containment of urine, and control of odor, product selection will be made by trial and error or will depend on product availability in the practice setting.

External Collection Devices. External collection devices such as condom catheters can be useful for management of UI in men because they contain urine and keep the skin dry. Although these devices are preferable to indwelling catheters, which have many side effects, adverse reactions do occur. Abrasion, dermatitis, ischemia, necrosis, edema, and maceration of the penis, as well as UTI, can be problems, especially as a result of improper or prolonged use (Ouslander, Greengold, and Chen, 1987a). External catheters need to be applied carefully and changed according to product recommendation and institutional or agency policy. Careful observation of the penile skin and the urine for adverse changes is mandatory.

Although a variety of external catheters is available, no comparative studies have been conducted. There is a need for studies to address the optimal length of time external catheters should be worn before changing and to compare the incidence of UTI and other complications between catheters and external and suprapubic catheters.

Acceptable external collecting devices for women are not widely available. Pieper and Cleland (1993) report that most products developed to date have never been marketed or sold. Still others have been removed from the market because of major problems of leakage and skin abrasions. The literature regarding these products consists of small descriptive studies performed outside of the United States (Pieper and Cleland, 1993). The results of two small studies performed in the United States are encouraging (Johnson, Muncie, O'Reilly, et al., 1990; Johnson, O'Reilly, and Warren, 1989); however, comparative or randomized studies have not been conducted. Thus, conclusions as to the efficiency and safety of these devices cannot be made.

Intermittent Catheterization

Intermittent catheterization appears to be preferable to the use of indwelling catheters for the management of urinary retention and overflow incontinence. (Strength of Evidence = B.)

Persons who have overflow incontinence can benefit from IC. Several studies indicate that IC is preferable to indwelling catheters for both men and women (Kuhan, Rist, and Zaech, 1991; Webb, Lawson, and Neal, 1990; Perkash and Giroux, 1993; Warren, 1990). However, the use of IC in the homebound patient may present considerable difficulty. Most studies have been conducted in young patients with spinal cord injuries. The section on Other Measures and Supportive Devices in Chapter 3 describes the various benefits and problems associated with IC.

Suprapubic Catheters

Suprapubic catheters may be an acceptable alternative for indwelling urethral catheters when patient choice or circumstances require the use of a bladder drainage device. (Strength of Evidence = B.)

Suprapubic catheterization may be an acceptable alternative to indwelling catheters or IC in some patients (Barnes, Shaw, Timoney, et al., 1993; Feneley, 1983; Hebel and Warren, 1990; Stower, Massey, and Feneley, 1989). Small descriptive studies indicate that suprapubic catheterization is a promising method of emptying the chronically full bladder. Large, randomized studies need to be conducted to compare the benefits and risks of this intervention with those of IC and indwelling catheters. In addition, studies should be performed on techniques that prevent the occurrence of complications.

Indwelling Catheters. The use of indwelling catheters should be avoided with few exceptions. They may be useful as comfort measures for the terminally ill, to avoid contamination of decubitus ulcers, and for management of UI in patients with inoperable obstruction that prevents bladder emptying. In Chapter 3, the section on Other Measures and Supportive Devices describes the serious problems associated with long-term use of indwelling catheters.

Skin Care

Recommended measures of cleansing the skin immediately before and after urine loss are helpful in preserving skin integrity. (Strength of Evidence = B.)

Some pads and garments may provide some protection from skin damage. (Strength of Evidence = C.)

Individuals with severe intractable incontinence are often immobile and at major risk for skin breakdown. No one would dispute the importance of good skin care and preventing skin breakdown, yet no randomized, controlled clinical trials have examined the methods most likely to achieve this goal. Recommendations about skin care are generally based on experience or made through marketing materials provided by product manufacturers (DeWitt, 1988; Fowler and Goupil, 1987; Klein, 1988). The most common directions to nurses are to keep the skin dry and keep the patient off any areas of skin breakdown.

Incontinence was noted as one of the risk factors for pressure ulcers in the AHCPR *Pressure Ulcers in Adults: Prediction and Prevention. Clinical Practice Guideline* (1992). The AHCPR guideline panels for Prediction and

Prevention of Pressure Ulcers in Adults (1992) and Treatment of Pressure Ulcers (1994) made several recommendations for the prevention of skin chafing and, ultimately, ulcer formation. Because of the lack of scientific evidence, these suggestions were based on expert opinion. Suggested preventive measures included regular inspection of the skin, gentle cleansing with a mild cleansing agent immediately after soiling, avoidance of force and friction during cleansing, use of absorptive briefs or pads, use of topical barriers to protect the skin from moisture, and minimizing skin injury caused by friction and shear through proper positioning, turning, and transfer techniques.

For a full discussion of skin breakdown, with recommendations for prevention and treatment of pressure ulcers, refer to the Clinical Practice Guidelines on pressure ulcers (Bergstrom, Bennett, Carlson, et al., 1994; Panel for the Prediction and Prevention of Pressure Ulcers in Adults, 1992).

Social and Organizational Milieu of UI

The social and organizational environment of the long-term care facilities can also impact on delivery of continence care. Training programs alone are not effective in changing practice routines from custodial to restorative (Campbell, Knight, Benson, et al., 1991; Colling, Ouslander, Hadley, et al., 1992). Even when well-planned programs exert a positive change on knowledge and attitude, nursing aide behavior may be unchanged (Lekan-Rutledge, Hogue, and Miller, 1992; Smyer, Brannon, and Cohn, 1992; Wagner and Colling, 1993). Long-term care staff are engaged in difficult work with few rewards. Burgio and Burgio (1990) noted in one study analyzing staff behavior that most staff time was spent in patient care activities. Certainly, before practice and management styles in long-term care can be changed, the current physical and social environment, including work patterns and numbers and type of staff, must be thoroughly explored. New nursing practice models such as the use of nurse practitioners and clinical nurse specialists have shown positive impact on resident health outcomes through improved care and decreased hospitalization of residents (Garrard, Kane, Radosevich, et al., 1990; Kane, Garrard, Skay, et al., 1989; Mezey, Lynaugh, and Cartier, 1989).

The few studies of UI in the dependent population in the community have focused on the burden experienced by unpaid caregivers, such as family members caring for dependent elderly persons with UI, and the effect of UI on the health and psychosocial adjustment of incontinent individuals. In all the studies, functional disability (physical, cognitive, or both) was associated with UI (Flaherty, Miller, and Col, 1992; Noelker, 1987; Ouslander, Zarit, Orr, et al., 1990). In a study of 299 family caregivers who cared for persons with UI, Noelker (1987) reported significantly more negative effects on family relationships than for caregivers of family members who were continent. However, nearly one-half of the caregivers of persons with UI stated that incontinence was not a problem for them. In another study of 148 caregivers of community-dwelling, chronically ill older persons, 75 percent of those who cared for incontinent family members found maintaining continence burdensome because of time spent in providing care, the care receiver's immobility, and lack of social supports (Flaherty, Miller, and Col, 1992). In a study of caregivers of community-dwelling dementia patients with UI, Ouslander, Zarit, Orr, et al. (1990) found that although incontinence was an important factor in many decisions to institutionalize elderly care receivers, UI was rarely the primary reason for nursing home placement, and other factors contributed more to perceived burden. Most of the caregivers indicated that they would be interested in education regarding the care of persons with UI if the sessions were provided in the home.

Although most persons can benefit from behavioral, pharmacologic, or surgical interventions for UI, many others cannot. Typically, these persons reside in long-term care facilities or are homebound and have cognitive or physical impairments that prevent them from learning or performing PME, bladder retraining, or other learned strategies to prevent urine leakage. They do not respond to regular toileting schedules. In addition, these dependent individuals often cannot tolerate or would not benefit from pharmacologic or surgical interventions.

In long-term care facilities, this population is largely cared for by non-professional nursing staff. Others are cared for at home most often by family members. Most of the research on UI has focused on reducing or eliminating leakage. Little attention has been given to how to provide the best care for those who do not respond to standard therapies. Studies to ascertain the most effective and efficient methods for specific situations and individual patients are needed to further advance optimal continence care. The care of persons who do not or cannot respond to available therapies must be addressed in randomized, clinically based studies. Currently, continence care for these persons is often based on personal opinion, manufacturers' claims, convenience of the caregiver, or cost of the products.

5 Education

Public Education

Increased efforts to inform and educate the public about incontinence are essential. (Strength of Evidence = C.)

The public should be aware that incontinence is not inevitable or shameful but is treatable or at least manageable. (Strength of Evidence = C.)

Patient education needs to be comprehensive and multidisciplinary so as to explain all management alternatives. (Strength of Evidence = C.)

More research is needed to test the effectiveness of patient education activities. (Strength of Evidence = C.)

UI has the stigma of a socially unacceptable condition because of public lack of knowledge, misconceptions, and intolerance. This leads to personal isolation, social embarrassment, and delays in seeking medical advice. The public needs to know that many therapy and management problems surround UI (Burton, 1984; Goldstein, Hawthorne, Engeberg, et al., 1992; Herzog, Fultz, Normolle, et al., 1989; Joseph Rowntree Foundation, 1991; Holst and Wilson, 1988; Lagace, Hansen, and Hickner, 1993; Norton, MacDonald, Sedgwick, et al., 1988; O'Brien, Austin, Sethi, et al., 1991; Thomas, Plymat, Blannin, et al., 1980). Since 1983, national and international groups have concluded that there is a lack of professional and public education about UI (Association for Continence Advice, 1993; Jeter and Gartley, 1994; Kings Fund, 1983; National Institutes of Health, 1990). In 1988, the National Institutes of Health (NIH) Consensus Development Conference on UI in adults concluded that there was a greater need for efforts to inform and educate the public about this common problem. However, specific education interventions were not designated. The research necessary to evaluate education programs specific for incontinence is lacking.

Since the 1988 NIH conference, public knowledge has increased somewhat through publication of the 1992 AHCPR guideline documents and the efforts of two self-help groups, Help for Incontinent People and the Simon Foundation for Continence. More than 1.3 million English-version and 125,000 Spanish-version AHCPR patient guides have been distributed since their 1992 release. The Continence Foundation offers public access to services and information in the United Kingdom. Education advocacy and support groups bridge the gap between the public, affected individuals, and the health care providers and provide multimedia resources, patient and health professional education, and patient referral services. Patients often turn to these groups for guidance and support. Letters to syndicated columnists Ann Landers and Abigail Van Buren (Dear Abby) about UI have also gained widespread reader attention. Product manufacturers are addressing UI through extensive media advertisements and publication of brochures, and in the United Kingdom some companies sponsor telephone helplines. One pharmaceutical company's pilot media program has attracted considerable public interest in seeking more information and medical advice on UI (Association for Continence Advice, 1993).

Healthy People 2000 recommends an increase in public education and self-help resources as well as a reduction in major activity limitations for the management of chronic conditions (U.S. Department of Health and Human Services, 1990). However, these efforts need to be increased so that the entire public is made aware that incontinence is neither inevitable nor shameful but instead treatable or at least manageable. The public should be encouraged to seek professional information and advice. Unfortunately, information alone is not enough to change behavior. A comprehensive and effective patient education program needs to determine what the patient wants to know as well as what the health care provider determines is necessary.

Two reports assess the information needs of the incontinent person (Jeter and Wagner, 1990; Moore and Saltmarche, 1993). An information-seeking instrument developed by Moore and Saltmarche has been tested for reliability and validity and will be used for data collection to guide patient education.

Because the problem of UI crosses all social, economic, racial, and gender lines, educational programs need to be diverse, person- or consumer-friendly, and understandable in a variety of media. Teaching should be a collaborative effort involving medical, nursing, and allied health care providers working with education and communication experts, and local, regional, and national government employers. Education should be individualized for each patient but also should include family and friends who may be involved in the patient's care. Sharing experiences and education in a nonthreatening atmosphere is a major technique of UI support groups and should be encouraged. Research to test educational effectiveness of these programs should be encouraged, developed, and evaluated, because specific research on UI patient teaching is lacking.

From available research, the main teaching goals that should be implemented are that (1) misconceptions about UI should be corrected, and information that incontinence can be helped should be disseminated to the widest possible audience; (2) patients with UI who seek health care need customized yet flexible patient teaching resources because of cultural, age, and educational differences; and (3) the learning experience should provide problem-solving and self-management skills that are integrated into daily living patterns. To accomplish these goals, a multimedia approach is needed that can provide information and education about UI misconceptions and management options at the learner's pace. Examples include use of public service announcements, public talk shows or interviews, health lectures, and toll-free telephone messages or helplines. Programs can be facilitated through pamphlets, booklets, audiotapes, videotapes, movies, slides, slide-tapes, film strips, computers, and interactive videodiscs. For example, an interactive laser disc program on treatment options for benign prostate hypertrophy led to a 60-percent drop in requests for prostatectomy (Borzo, 1994). The applicability of such a program for incontinence should be tested. It is essential that teaching effectiveness be evaluated because instructing patients is insufficient (Garding, Kerr, and Bay, 1988).

Similarly, knowledge on ways to prevent UI is lacking. Examples of possible preventive maneuvers include teaching women about gestational and postpartum PME, and teaching both men and women about scheduled voiding and proper bladder-emptying techniques. Other health promotion models describe primary prevention mechanisms including education programs regarding estrogen use to treat atrophic vaginitis, postmenopausal changes of the genitourinary tract, and the elimination of fluids with diuretic effects (Palmer, 1994). When the public learns to better manage UI and to seek early treatment, the personal, social, psychological, and economic costs of the condition will decrease.

Professional Education

Education about UI evaluation and treatment should be included in the basic curricula of undergraduate and graduate training programs of all health care providers. Continuing education programs on UI should be offered to all health care providers. (Strength of Evidence = C.)

Education about UI for professionals, paraprofessionals, and survey teams is urgently needed. First and foremost, information about UI should be included in the curricula of undergraduate and graduate health care professional schools. Schools of nursing and physical therapy and for physician assistants should consider educating specialists on incontinence care who can then serve as expert advisers to other health care providers regionally, on the State level, in teaching hospitals, and in every nursing home.

To increase practitioners' knowledge of UI, continuing education courses should focus on the types of incontinence and on appropriate, state-of-the-art diagnostic techniques and treatments (Morishita, Uman, and Pierson, 1994). Professionals most likely to provide care to UI patients should be encouraged to attend these courses. Education on UI should also be part of the training programs for paraprofessional students, such as licensed vocational nurses, practice nurses' aides, and auxiliary workers in the community. Because UI is a major problem in long-term care settings, special emphasis should be directed to encouraging alliances among all professions responsible for the care of persons with UI. In this setting, education may need to be geared to the different levels of nursing personnel. Palmer (1995) in a survey about nurses' knowledge and beliefs about continence interventions in one nursing home found differences between attributions of cause of UI between LPNs and RNs, indicating a need for continued education.

A survey of physicians in an Oklahoma demonstration project revealed that

17 percent of physicians had seen or read the 1992 AHCPR guideline on UI. This group included internists (113), obstetricians and gynecologists (134), family practitioners (115), and urologists (14) (McFall, Yerkes, Belzer, et al., 1994). Many physicians do not discuss nonsurgical therapy alternatives with their patients because they have a selection bias. UI should be included in the curricula along with practical applications and demonstrations that the majority of UI patients can be managed in primary care settings.

Major nursing organizations recognize the significance of UI and the vital role of nursing professionals. Plans are ongoing for development of continence care nursing practice guidelines. Emulation of the United Kingdom Continence Advisors program is a plausible solution but necessitates government involvement. A number of education organizations exist in the United Kingdom that provide training and education and whose members work in collaboration with other health care providers (Association for Incontinence Advice, 1993). Education and competency training for nurse practitioners in UI assessment and management can duplicate the Continence Advisors program. Conferences similar to the Multispecialty Nursing Conference on UI (held in Phoenix, Arizona, January 1994) can offer indepth education and provide training on technical skills so that these individuals can become productive and valued members of the UI team.

UI outcome measures need to be developed so that nursing home surveyors are better able to assess the effectiveness of interventions for UI in this setting.

References

Abbassian A. Colpovesical neck suspension for the correction of female stress urinary incontinence. J Urol 1989;142:95–6.

Abrams P, Blaivas JG, Stanton SL, Andersen JT. Standardization of terminology of lower urinary tract function. Neurourol Urodyn 1988;7:403–27.

Adams C, Lorish C, Cushing C, Willis E. Anatomical urinary stress incontinence in women with rheumatoid arthritis: its frequency and coping strategies. Arthr Care Res 1994 Jun;7(2):97–103.

Alloussi S, Loew F, Mast GJ, Alzin H, Wolf D. Treatment of detrusor instability of the urinary bladder by selective sacral blockade. Br J Urol 1984;56:464.

Andersson KE. Current concepts in the treatment of disorders of micturition. Drugs 1988;35(1):477–94.

Appell RA. Collagen injection therapy for urinary incontinence. Urol Clin North Am 1994;21(1):177–82.

Appell RA. Techniques and results in the implantation of the artificial urinary sphincter in women with type III stress urinary incontinence by a vaginal approach. Neurourol Urodyn 1988;134:476.

Appell RA, Baum N. Neurogenic bladder in diabetes. Pract Diabetol 1990;9(4):1–4.

Araki T, Takamoto H, Hara T, Fujimoto H, Yoshida M, Katayama Y. The loop-loosening procedure for urination difficulties after Stamey suspension of the vesical neck. J Urol 1990;144:319–23.

Ashken MH. Follow-up results with the Stamey operation for stress incontinence of urine. Br J Urol 1990;65:168–9.

Association for Continence Advice. Guidelines for continence care. London: Association for Continence Advice; 1993. p. 20.

Awad SA, Gajewski JB, Katz NO, Acker-Roy K. Final diagnosis and therapeutic implications of mixed symptoms of urinary incontinence in women. Urology 1992;34:352–7.

Baigis-Smith J, Smith DAJ, Rose M, Newman DK. Managing urinary incontinence in community-residing elderly persons. Gerontologist 1989;29(2):229–33.

Baker DI, Bice TW. The influence of urinary incontinence on publicly financed home care services to low-income elderly people. Gerontologist 1995;35(3):360–9.

Baker KR, Drutz HP. Age as a risk factor in major genitourinary surgery. Can J Surg 1992;35:188–91.

Barnes DG, Shaw PJR, Timoney AG, Tsokos N. Management of the neuropathic bladder by suprapubic catheterisation. Br J Urol 1993;72:169–72.

Beck RP, Arnusch D, King C. Results in treating 210 patients with detrusor overactivity incontinence of urine. Am J Obstet Gynecol 1976;125:593–6.

Beck RP, McCormick S, Nordstrom L. A 25 year experience with 519 anterior colporrhaphy procedures. Obstet Gynecol 1991;78:1011.

Beck RP, McCormick S, Nordstrom L. The fascia lata sling procedure for treating recurrent genuine stress incontinence of urine. Obstet Gynecol 1988;72:699–703.

Beck RP, Thomas EA, Maughan GB. Surgical results in the treatment of pressure equalization stress incontinence. Am J Obstet Gynecol 1968;100:483–9.

Beckingham IJ, Wemyss-Holden G, Lawrence WT. Long term follow-up of women treated with periurethral teflon injections for stress incontinence. Br J Urol 1992;69:580–3.

Benbow S, Sangster G, Barer D. Incontinence after stroke [letter comment]. Lancet 1991 Dec 21–28;338(8782–3):1602–3.

Benderev TV. Anchor fixation and other modifications of endoscopic bladder neck suspensions. Urology 1992;40:409–18.

Benson JT. Gynecologic and urodynamic evaluation of women with urinary incontinence. Obstet Gynecol 1985;66:691–4.

Benson JT, Agosta A, McClellan E. Evaluation of a minimal-incision pubovaginal suspension as an adjunct to other pelvic floor surgery. Obstet Gynecol 1990;75:844.

Benson JT, Sumners JE. Ultrasound evaluation of female urinary incontinence. Int Urogynecol J 1990;1(1):7–11.

Bent AE, Sand PK, Ostergard DR, Brubaker L. Transvaginal electrical stimulation in the treatment of genuine stress incontinence and detrusor instability. Int Urogynecol J 1993;4:9–13.

Benvenuti F, Caputo GM, Bandinelli S, Mayer F, Biagini C, Sommavilla A. Re-educative treatment of female genuine stress incontinence. Am J Phys Ther 1987;66:155–68.

Berg S. Polytef augmentation urethroplasty. Arch Surg 1973;107:379.

Bergman A, Ballard CA, Koonings PP. Comparison of three different surgical procedures for genuine stress incontinence: prospective randomized study. Am J Obstet Gynecol 1989;160:1102–6.

Bergman A, Koonings PP, Ballard CA. Negative q-tip test as a risk factor for failed incontinence surgery in women. J Reprod Med 1989a;34:193–4.

Bergman A, Koonings PP, Ballard CA. Primary stress urinary incontinence and pelvic relaxation: prospective randomized comparison of three different operations. Am J Obstet Gynecol 1989c;161:97–101.

Bergman A, Koonings PP, Ballard CA. Proposed management of low urethral pressure type of genuine stress urinary incontinence. Gynecol Obstet Invest 1989b;27:155–9.

Bergmann S, Eriksen BC. Anal electrostimulation in urinary incontinence. Urol Int 1986;41:411–7.

Bergstrom N, Bennett MA, Carlson CE, et al. Treatment of pressure ulcers. Clinical practice guideline, no. 15. AHCPR Publication No. 95-0652. Rockville (MD): U.S. Department of Health and Human Services. Public Health Service, Agency for Health Care Policy and Research; December 1994.

Bhatia NN, Bergman A. Modified Burch versus Pereyra retropubic urethropexy for stress urinary incontinence. Obstet Gynecol 1985a;66(2):255–61.

Bhatia NN, Bergman A. Pessary test in women with urinary incontinence. Obstet Gynecol 1985b;65:220.

Bjork DT, Pelletier LL, Tight RR. Urinary tract infections with antibiotic resistant organisms in catheterized nursing home patients. Infect Control 1984;5(4):173–6.

Blackford HN, Murray K, Stephenson TP, Mundy AR. Results of transvesical infiltration of the pelvic plexuses with phenol in 116 patients. Br J Urol 1984;56:647.

Blacklock, NJ. Catheters and urethral strictures. Br J Urol 1986;58:475–8.

Blaivas JG. Pathophysiology of lower urinary tract dysfunction. Urol Clin North Am 1985;12:215–24.

Blaivas JG, Labib AB, Michalik SJ, Zayed AAH. Cystometric response to propantheline in detrusor hyperreflexia therapeutic implications. J Urol 1980;124(2):259–62.

Blowman C, Pickles C, Emery S, Creates V, Towell L, Blackburn N, Doyle N, Walkden B. Prospective double blind controlled trial of intensive physiotherapy with and without stimulation of the pelvic floor in treatment of genuine stress incontinence. Physiotherapy 1991;77(10):661–4.

Bo K, Hagen RM, Kvarstein B, Jorgensen J, Larsen S. Pelvic floor muscle exercises for the treatment of female stress urinary incontinence III. Effects of two different degrees of pelvic floor muscle exercises. Neurourol Urodyn 1990;9(5):489–502.

Bo K, Maehlum S, Oseid S, Larsen S. Prevalence of stress urinary incontinence among physically active and sedentary female students. Scand J Sports Sci 1989;11(3):113–6.

Borzo G. CIGNA gives new life to patient empowerment initiative. American Medical News. September 19, 1994: 1, 8.

Boscia JA, Kobasa WD, Abrutyn E, Levison ME, Kaplan AM, Kaye D. Lack of association between bacteriuria and symptoms in the elderly. Am J Med 1986;81:979–82.

Bosman G, Vierhout ME, Huikeshoven JM. A modified Raz bladder neck suspension operation. Acta Obstet Gynecol Scand 1993;72:47–9.

Boulter CS, editor. Minimum data set and reference manual. Natick (MA): Eliot Press; 1993.

Bramble FJ. The treatment of adult enuresis and urge incontinence by enterocystoplasty. Br J Urol 1982;54(6):693–6.

Branch LG, Walker LA, Wetle TT, DuBeau CE, Resnick NM. Urinary incontinence knowledge among community-dwelling people 65 years of age and older. J Am Geriatr Soc 1994;42(12):1257–62.

Breakwell SL, Walker SN. Differences in physical health, social interaction, and personal adjustment between continent and incontinent homebound aged women. J Commun Health Nurs 1988;5(1):19–31.

Bridges N, Denning J, Olah KS, Aorrar DJ. A prospective trial comparing interferential therapy and treatment using cones in patients with symptoms of stress incontinence. Neurourol Urodyn 1988;7(3):267–8.

Brieger G, Korda A. The effect of obesity on the outcome of successful surgery for genuine stress incontinence. Aust N Z J Obstet Gynaecol 1992;32:71–2.

Brink, C. Absorbent pads, garments and management strategies. J Am Geriatr Soc 1990;38:363–73.

Brink C. Absorbent products and collecting devices: the patient with intractable incontinence: managing incontinence in elderly dependent institutionalized and community dwelling persons [abstract]. Presented at conference; 1994 Mar; Atlanta, GA.

Brink C, Wells JJ, Diokno AC. Urinary incontinence in women. Public Health Nurs 1987;4(2):114–9.

Brito CG, Mulcahy JJ, Mitchell ME, Adams MC. Use of a double cuff AMS800 urinary sphincter for severe stress incontinence. J Urol 1993;149:283–5.

Brocklehurst JC, Hickey DS, Davies I, Kennedy AP, Morris JA. A new urethral catheter. BMJ 1988 June;296:1691–3.

Bryans FE. Marlex gauze hammock sling operation with Cooper's ligament attachment in the management of recurrent urinary stress incontinence. Am J Obstet Gynecol 1979;133:292.

Bump RC, Hurt WG, Fantl A, Wyman JF. Assessment of Kegel pelvic exercise performance after brief verbal instruction. Am J Obstet Gynecol 1991;165:322–9.

Bump RC, McClish DM. Cigarette smoking and pure genuine stress incontinence of urine. A comparison of risk factors and determinants between smokers and non-smokers. Am J Obstet Gynecol 1994;170(2):579–82.

Burgio K, Whitehead WE, Engel BT. Urinary incontinence in the elderly: bladder-sphincter biofeedback and toileting skills training. Ann Intern Med 1985;104:507–15.

Burgio KL, Engel BT. Biofeedback-assisted behavioral training for elderly men and women. J Am Geriatr Soc 1990;38(3):338–40.

Burgio KL, Ives DG, Locher JL, Arena VC. Treatment seeking for urinary incontinence in adults. J Am Geriatr Soc 1994;42(2):208–12.

Burgio KL, Matthews KA, Engel BT. Prevalence, incidence and correlates of urinary incontinence in healthy, middle-aged women. J Urol 1991;146:1255–9.

Burgio KL, Robinson JC, Engel BT. The role of biofeedback in Kegel exercise training for stress urinary incontinence. Am J Obstet Gynecol 1986;154(1):58–64.

Burgio KL, Stutzman RE, Engel BT. Behavioral training for post-prostatectomy urinary incontinence. J Urol 1989;141:303–6.

Burgio LD, Burgio K. Institutional staff training and management: a review of the literature and a model for geriatric long term care facilities. Int J Aging Hum Devel 1990;30:287–302.

Burgio LD, Engel BT, McCormick KA, Hawkins AM, Scheve A. Behavioral treatment for UI in elderly inpatients: initial attempts to modify prompting and toileting procedures. Behav Ther 1988;19:345–57.

Burgio LD, McCormick KA, Scheve AS, Engel BT, Hawkins A, Leahy E. The effects of changing prompted voiding schedules in the treatment of incontinence in nursing home residents. J Am Geriatr Soc 1994;42(3):315–20.

Burns P, Nochajski T, Pranifoff K. Predictors of incontinence in elderly women [abstract]. Proceedings of the International Continence Society, 23rd Annual Meeting. Neurourol Urodyn 1993;12(4):432–4.

Burns PA, Marecki MA, Dittmar SS, Bullough B. Kegel's exercises with biofeedback therapy for treatment of stress incontinence. Nurse Pract 1985;28–46.

Burns PA, Pranifoff K, Nochajski T, Desotelle P, Harwood MK. Treatment of stress incontinence with pelvic floor exercises and biofeedback. J Am Geriatr Soc 1990;38(3):341–4.

Burns PA, Pranifoff K, Nochajski TH, Hadley EC, Levy KJ, Ory MG. A comparison of effectiveness of biofeedback and pelvic muscle exercise treatment of stress-incontinence in older community-dwelling women. J Gerontol 1993 Jul;48(4):167–74.

Burton J, Pearce L, Burgio KL, Engel BT, Whitehead WE. Behavioral training for urinary incontinence in elderly, ambulatory patients. J Am Geriatr Soc 1988;36(8):693–8.

Burton JR. Managing urinary incontinence—a common geriatric problem. Geriatrics 1984;39(10):46–62.

Cammu H, Van Nylen J, Derde MP, DeBruyne R, Amy JJ. Pelvic physiotherapy in genuine stress incontinence. Urology 1991 Oct;38(4):332–7.

Campbell EB, Knight M, Benson M, Colling J. Effect of an incontinence training program on nursing home staff's knowledge, attitudes, and behaviors. Gerontologist 1991;31:788–94.

Caputo RM, Bensen JT, McClellan E. Intravaginal maximal electrical stimulation in the treatment of urinary incontinence. J Rep Med 1993 Sep;38(9):667–71.

Cardozo LD, Stanton SL. An objective comparison of the effects of parenterally administered drugs in patients suffering from detrusor instability. J Urol 1979;122:58.

Cardozo LD, Stanton SL, Robinson H, Holer D. Evaluation of flurbiprofen in detrusor instability. BMJ 1980;280:281–2.

Castleden CM, Duffin HM, Asher MJ, Yeomanson CW. Factors influencing outcome in elderly patients with urinary incontinence and detrusor instability. Age Ageing 1985;14:303–7.

Castleden CM, Duffin HM, Gulati RS. Double-blind study of imipramine and placebo for incontinence due to bladder instability. Age Ageing 1986;15(5):299–303.

Castleden CM, Duffin HM, Millar AW. Dicyclomine hydrochloride in detrusor instability: a controlled clinical pilot study. J Clin Exp Gerontol 1987;9(4):265–70.

Castleden NS, Duffin HM, Mitchell EP. The effects of physiotherapy on stress incontinence. Age Ageing 1984;13:235–7.

Cella M. The nursing costs of urinary incontinence in a nursing home population. Nurs Clin North Am 1988;23:159–68.

Chapple CR, Parkhouse H, Gardener C, Milroy EJ. Double-blind, placebo-controlled, crossover study of flavoxate in the treatment of idiopathic detrusor instability. Br J Urol 1990 Nov;66(5):491–4.

Claes H, Stroobants D. Pulmonary migration following periurethral polytetrafluoroethylene injection for urinary incontinence. J Urol 1989;142:821–2.

Cobb OE, Ragde H. Simplified correction of female stress incontinence. J Urol 1978;120:418–20.

Colling J, Ouslander J, Hadley BJ, Eisch J, Campbell E. The effects of patterned urge response toileting (PURT) on urinary incontinence among nursing home residents. J Am Geriatr Soc 1992;40:135–41.

Colling JC, Owen TR, McCreedy MR. Urine volumes and voiding patterns among incontinent nursing home residents. Residents at highest risk for dehydration are often the most difficult to track. Geriatr Nurs 1994;15(4):188–92.

Collste L, Lindskog M. Phenylpropanolamine in treatment of female stress urinary incontinence: a double-blind placebo-controlled study in 24 patients. Urodynamics 1987 Oct;30(4):398–403.

Coombes GM, Millard RJ. The accuracy of portable ultrasound scanning in the measurement of residual urine volume. J Urol 1994;152:2083–5.

Corrie D, Rodriguez FR, Thompson IM. Periurethral polytetrafluoroethylene injections for post-prostatectomy incontinence. Mil Med 1989 Aug;154(9):442–4.

Cox AG, Hukins DWL, Sutton HM. Infection of catheterized patients: Bacterial colonization of encrusted Foley catheters. Urol Res 1989;17:349–52.

Creason NS, Grybowski JA, Burgener S, Whippo C, Yeo SA, Richardson B. Prompted voiding therapy for urinary incontinence in aged female nursing home residents. J Adv Nurs 1989;14:120–6.

Crieghton AM, Stanton SL. Caffeine: does it affect your bladder? Br J Urol 1990;66:613–4.

Curling M, Broome G, Gendry WF. How accurate is urine cytology? J Roy Soc Med 1986;79:336–8.

Davila GW, Osterman KV. The bladder neck support prosthesis: a nonsurgical approach to stress incontinence in adult women. Am J Obstet Gynecol 1994;71(1):206–11.

Davis KM, Minaker KL. Disorders of fluid balance: dehydration and hyponatremia. In: Hazzard WK, Bierman EL, Blass JP, Ettinger WH, Walter JB, editors. Principles of geriatric medicine and gerontology. 3rd ed. New York: McGraw Hill; 1994.

Deane AM, English P, Hehir M, Williams JP, Worth PHL. Teflon injection in stress incontinence. Br J Urol 1985;57:78.

Deppe G, Castro-Marin A, Nachamie R, Adamsons K. Urethral fascial sling operation for repair of urinary stress incontinence: ten cases at the Mount Sinai Hospital from 1972–1973. Mt Sinai J Med 1978;45:166.

Dequeker J. Drug treatment of urinary incontinence in the elderly. Controlled trial with vasopressin and propantheline bromide. Gerontol Clin 1965;7(5):311–7.

DeWitt S. Skin conditions common to the urology patient. J Urol Nurs 1988;74(4):501–4.

Dijkman GA, Friese S. Vesical-urethral sustaining for recurrent urinary stress incontinence using the Stamey-Pereyra technique. Acta Urol Belg 1984;52:302–5.

Diokno AC. Diagnostic categories of incontinence and the role of urodynamic testing. J Am Geriatr Soc 1990;38(3):300–5.

Diokno AC, Brock BM, Brown HB, Herzog AR. Prevalence of urinary incontinence and other urologic symptoms in the non-institutionalized elderly. J Urol 1986;136:1022–5.

Diokno AC, Brock BM, Herzog AR, Bromberg J. Medical correlates of urinary incontinence in the elderly. Urology 1990;36:129–38.

Diokno AC, Brown MB, Brock BM, Herzog AR, Normolle DP. Clinical and cystometric characteristics of continent and incontinent noninstitutionalized elderly. J Urol 1988;140:567–71.

Diokno AC, Hollander JB, Alderson TP. Artificial urinary sphincter for recurrent female urinary incontinence: indications and results. J Urol 1987;138:778.

Diokno AC, Koff SA, Anderson W. Combined cystometry and perineal electromyography in the diagnosis and treatment of neurogenic urinary incontinence. J Urol 1976;115(2):161–3.

Diokno AC, Normolle DP, Brown MB, Herzog AR. Urodynamic tests for female geriatric urinary incontinence. Urology 1990;36(5):431–9.

Diokno AC, Sonda LP, Hollander JB, Lapides J. Fate of patients started on clean intermittent self-catheterization therapy 10 years ago. J Urol 1983;129:1120–2.

Diokno AC, Vinson RK, McGillicuddy J. Treatment of the severe uninhibited neurogenic bladder by selective sacral rhizotomy. J Urol 1977;118:299.

Diokno AC, Wells TJ, Brink CA. Comparison of self-reported voided volume with cystometric bladder capacity. J Urol 1987;137(4):698–700.

Dougherty MC, Abrams R, McKey PL. An instrument to assess the dynamic characteristics of the circumvaginal musculature. Nurs Res 1986;35:202–6.

Dougherty M, Bishop K, Mooney R, Gimotty P, Williams B. Graded pelvic muscle exercise. Effect on stress urinary incontinence. J Reprod Med 1993 Sep;39(9):684–91.

Duncan HJ, Nurse DE, Mundy AR. Role of the artificial urinary sphincter in the treatment of stress incontinence in women. Br J Urol 1992;69:141–3.

Dwyer PL, Teele JS. Prazosin: a neglected cause of genuine stress incontinence. Obstet Gynecol 1992;79:117–21.

Eckford SD, Abrams P. Para-urethral collagen implantation for female stress incontinence. Br J Urol 1991;68:586–9.

Ek A, Andersson KE, Gullberg B, Ulmsten U. Effects of oestradiol and combined norephedrine and oestradiol treatment on female stress incontinence. Zentralbl Gynakol 1980;102(15):839–44.

Ek A, Andersson KE, Gullberg B, Ulmsten U. The effects of long-term treatment with norephedrine on stress incontinence and urethral closure pressure profile. Scand J Urol Nephrol 1978;12(2):105–10.

Elia G, Bergman A. Pelvic muscle exercises: when do they work? Obstet Gynecol 1993 Feb;81(2):283–6.

Elliott TSJ, Gopal Rao G, Reid L, Woodhouse K. Long-term urethral catheterisation in the elderly [letter]. BMJ 1987 April;294:1095–6.

Engel BT, Burgio LD, McCormick KA, Hawkins AM, Scheve AS, Leahy E. Behavioral treatment of incontinence in the long-term care setting. J Am Geriatr Soc 1990;38:361–3.

Eriksen BC. Electrostimulation of the pelvic floor in female urinary incontinence. Acta Obstet Gynecol Scand 1990;69:359–60.

Eriksen BC, Bergmann S, Eik-Nes SH. Maximal electrostimulation of the pelvic floor in female idiopathic detrusor instability and urge incontinence. Neurourol Urodyn 1989;8:219–30.

Eriksen BC, Bergmann S, Mjolnerod OK. Effect of anal electrostimulation with the "Incontan" device in women with urinary incontinence. Br J Obstet Gynaecol 1987;94:147–56.

Eriksen BC, Eik-Nes SH. Long-term electrical stimulation of the pelvic floor: primary therapy in female stress incontinence? Urol Int 1989;44:90–5.

Eriksen BC, Hagen B, Eik-Nes SH, Molne K, Mjolnerod OK, Romslo I. Long-term effectiveness of the Burch colposuspension in female urinary stress incontinence. Acta Obstet Gynecol Scand 1990;69:45–50.

Eriksen BC, Mjolnerod OK. Changes in urodynamic measurements after successful anal electrostimulation in female urinary incontinence. Br J Urol 1987;59:45–9.

Esa A, Kiwamoto H, Sugiyama T, Park YC, Kaneko S, Kurita T. Functional electrical stimulation in the management of incontinence: studies of urodynamics. Int Urol Nephrol 1991;23:135–41.

Evans LK, Strumpf NE. Myths about elder restraint. Image 1990;22:124–9.

Ewing R, Bultitude MI, Shuttleworth KED. Subtrigonal phenol injection for urge incontinence secondary to detrusor instability in females. Br J Urol 1982;54:689.

Fall M, Ahlstrom K, Carlsson CA, Ek A, Erlandson BE, Frankenberg S, Mattiasson A. Contelle: pelvic floor stimulator for female stress-urge incontinence. Urology 1986;27(3):282–7.

Fall M, Erlandson BE, Pettersson S. Evaluation of history and simple supine cystometry as a preoperative test in stress urinary incontinence. Acta Obstet Gynecol Scand 1984;63:241–4.

Fantl JA, Cardozo L, McClish DK, Hormones and Urogenital Therapy Committee. Estrogen therapy in the management of urinary incontinence in postmenopausal women: a meta-analysis: first report of the hormones and urogenital therapy committee. Obstet Gynecol 1994;83:12–8.

Fantl JA, Smith PJ, Schneider V, Hunt WG, Dunn LJ. Fluid weight uroflowmetry in women. Am J Obstet Gynecol 1983;145(8):1017–24.

Fantl JA, Wyman JF, McClish DK, Bump RC. Urinary incontinence in community-dwelling women: clinical, urodynamic and severity characteristics. Am J Obstet Gynecol 1990;162(4):946–51.

Fantl JA, Wyman JF, McClish DK, Harkins SW, Elswick RK, Taylor JR, et al. Efficacy of bladder training in older women with urinary incontinence. JAMA 1991;265(5):609–13.

Feneley R. The management of female incontinence by suprapubic catheterization, with or without urethral closure. Br J Urol 1983 May;55:203–7.

Fenn N, Conn IG, German KA, Stephenson TP. Complications of clam enterocystoplasty with particular reference to urinary tract infection. Br J Urol 1992;69:366–8.

Ferguson K, McKey PL, Bishop KR, Kloen P, Verheul JB, Dougherty MC. Stress urinary incontinence: effect of pelvic muscle exercise. Obstet Gynecol 1990;73:671–5.

Ferriani RA, de Sa MDA, de Moura MC, Charaffedine MN, de Freitas Junior AH. Ureteral blockage as a complication of Burch colposuspension: report of 6 cases. Gynecol Obstet Invest 1990;29:239–40.

Ferrie BG, Smith JS, Logan D, Lyle R, Paterson PJ. Experience with bladder training in 65 patients. Br J Urol 1984;56:482–4.

Finlay OE, Bayles TB, Rosen C, Milling J. Effects of chair design, age and cognitive status on mobility. Age Ageing 1983;12(4):329–35.

Fischer-Rasmussen W, Hansen RI, Stage P. Predictive values of diagnostic tests in the evaluation of female urinary stress incontinence. Acta Obstet Gynecol Scand 1986;65:291–4.

Flaherty JH, Miller DK, Col RM. Impact on caregivers of supporting urinary function in non institutionalized chronically ill seniors. Gerontologist 1992;32(4):541–5.

Flynn L, Cell P, Luisi E. Effectiveness of pelvic exercises in reducing urge incontinence. J Gerontol Nurs 1994;20(5):23–7.

Foldspang A, Mommsen S, Lam FW, Elving L. Parity as a correlate of adult female urinary incontinence prevalence. J Epidemiol Community Health 1992;46:595–600.

Folstein MF, Folstein S, McHugh PR. Mini-Mental State: a practical method for grading the cognitive state of patients for the health care provider. J Psych Res 1975;12:189–98.

Fonda A. Improving management of urinary incontinence in geriatric centers and nursing homes. Victorian Geriatrician Peer Review Group. Austral Clin Rev (Sydney) 1990;10(2):66–71.

Fonda D, Brimage PJ, D'Astoli M. Simple screening for urinary incontinence in the elderly: comparison of simple and multichannel cystometry. Urology 1993 Nov;42(5):536–40.

Fossberg E, Beisland HO, Lundgren RA. Stress incontinence in females: treatment with phenylpropanolamine: a urodynamic and pharmacological evaluation. Urol Int 1983;38(5):293–9.

Fossberg E, Sorensen S, Ruutu M, Bakke A, Stien R, Henriksen L, Kinn AC. Maximal electrical stimulation in the treatment of unstable detrusor and urge incontinence. Eur Urol 1990;18:120–3.

Foster MC, O'Reilly PH. Early experience of the Gittes "no-incision" pubovaginal suspension for stress urinary incontinence. Br J Urol 1989;64:590–3.

Fowler JE. Experience with suprapubic vesicourethral suspension and endoscopic suspension of the vesical neck for stress urinary incontinence in females. Surg Gynecol Obstet 1986;162:437–41.

Fowler EL, Goupil D. Managing an incontinence problem: assessment, plan, and products. J Urol Nurs (Special Ed) 1987;282:288.

Francis LN, Sand PK, Hamrang K, Ostergard DR. A urodynamic appraisal of success and failure after retropubic urethropexy. J Reprod Med 1987;32:693–6.

Ganabathi K, Abrams P, Mundy AR, et al. Stamey-Martius procedure for severe genuine stress incontinence. Br J Urol 1992;69:34–7.

Garding BS, Kerr JC, Bay K. Effectiveness of a program of information and support for myocardial infarction patients recovering at home. Heart Lung 1988;17:355–62.

Garrard J, Kane RL, Radosevich DM, Skay CL. Impact of geriatric nurse practitioners on nursing home residents functional status, satisfaction, and discharge outcomes. Med Care 1990;38(3):361–3.

Gaum L, Ricciotti NA, Fair WR. Endoscopic bladder neck suspension for stress urinary incontinence. J Urol 1984;132:1119–21.

George NK, Russel GL. Clam ileocystoplasty. Br J Urol 1991;68:487–9.

Gilja I, Radej M, Kovacic M, Parazajder J. Conservative treatment of female stress incontinence with imipramine. J Urol 1984;132(5):909–11.

Gittes RF, Laughlin KR. No incision pubovaginal suspension for stress incontinence. J Urol 1987;138:568–70.

Gleason DM, Reilly RJ, Bottaccini MR, Pierce MJ. The urethral continence zone and its relation to stress incontinence. J Urol 1974;112(1):81–8.

Godec CJ. Timed voiding: a useful tool in the treatment of urinary incontinence. Urology 1994;23(1):97–100.

Goldstein I, Wise GJ, Tancer ML. A vesicovaginal fistula and intravesical foreign body. Am J Obstet Gynecol 1990;163:589–91.

Goldstein M, Hawthorne ME, Engeberg S, McDowell BJ, Burgio KL. Urinary incontinence: why people do not seek help. J Gerontol Nurs 1992;18(4):15–20.

Goodno JA, Powers TW. Modified retropubic cysturethropexy II. Am J Obstet Gynecol 1992;166:1678–82.

Grahn D, Norman DC, White ML, Cantreel M, Yoshikawa TT. Validity of urinary catheter specimen for diagnosis of urinary tract infection in the elderly. Arch Intern Med 1985 Oct;145:1858–60.

Green DF, McGuire EJ, Lytton B. A comparison of endoscopic suspension of the vesical neck versus anterior urethropexy for the treatment of stress urinary incontinence. J Urol 1986;136:1205–7.

Green RJ, Laycock J. Objective methods for evaluation of interferential therapy in the treatment of incontinence. IEEE Trans Biomed Eng 1990;37:615–23.

Griffith-Jones MD, Abrams H. The Stamey endoscopic bladder neck suspension in the elderly. Br J Urol 1990;65:170–2.

Grimby A, Milsom I, Molander U, Wiklund I, Ekelund P. The influence of urinary incontinence on the quality of life of elderly women. Age Ageing 1993 Mar;22(2):82–9.

Gundian JC, Barrett DM, Parulkar BG. Mayo Clinic experience with use of the AMS 800 artificial urinary sphincter for urinary incontinence following radical prostatectomy. J Urol 1989;142:1459.

Hahn I, Sommar S, Fall M. A comparative study of pelvic floor training and electrical stimulation for the treatment of female stress urinary incontinence. Neurourol Urodyn 1991;10:545–54.

Harke JM, Richgels K. Barriers to implementing a continence program in nursing homes. Clin Nurs Res 1992;1:158–68.

Harris T. Aging in the eighties: prevalence and impact of urinary problems in individuals age 65 years and over. Washington, DC: Department of Health and Human Services, National Center for Health Statistics, No. 121, August 27, 1986.

Harrison GL, Memel DS. Urinary incontinence in women: its prevalence and its management in a health promotion clinic. Br J Gen Pract 1994 Apr;44(381):149–52.

Harrison SCW, Brown C, O'Boyle PJ. Periurethral teflon for stress urinary incontinence: medium-term results. Br J Urol 1993;71:25–7.

Haylen BT, Frazer MI, MacDonald JH. Assessing the effectiveness of different urinary catheters in emptying the bladder: an application of transvaginal ultrasound. Br J Urol 1989;64(4):353–6.

Health Care Financing Administration. Long term care facility Resident Assessment Instrument (RAI) user's manual for use with version 2.0 of the Health Care Financing Administration's Minimum Data Set, Resident Assessment Protocols, and Utilization Guidelines. Baltimore (MD): Health Care Financing Administration; 1995.

Hebel JR, Warren JW. The use of urethral, condom and suprapubic catheters in aged nursing home patients. J Am Geriatr Soc 1990;38:777–84.

Heller BR, Whitehead WE, Johnson LD. Incontinence. J Gerontol Nurs 1989;15(5):16–23.

Henalla SM, Kirwan P, Castleden CM, Hutchens CJ, Breeson AJ. The effect of pelvic floor exercises in the treatment of genuine urinary stress incontinence in women at two hospitals. Br J Obstet Gynaecol 1988;95:602–6.

Herzog AR, Fultz NH, Normolle DP, Brock BM, Diokno AC. Methods used to manage urinary incontinence by older adults in the community. J Am Geriatr Soc 1989;37(4):339–47.

Hilton P. A clinical and urodynamic study comparing the Stamey bladder neck suspension and suburethral sling procedures in the treatment of genuine stress incontinence. Br J Obstet Gynaecol 1989;96:213–20.

Hilton P, Stanton SL. Urethral pressure measurement by micro-transducer: the results in symptom-free women and in those with genuine stress incontinence. Br J Obstet Gynaecol 1983;90:919.

Hilton P, Tweddell AL, Mayne C. Oral and intravaginal estrogens alone and in combination with alpha-adrenergic stimulation in genuine stress incontinence. Int Urogynecol J 1990;1(2):80–6.

Hodgkinson CP, Drukker BH. Infravesical nerve resection for detrusor dyssynergia. Acta Obstet Gynecol Scand 1977;56:401.

Holmes DM, Montz FJ, Stanton SL. Oxybutynin versus propantheline in the management of detrusor instability: a patient-regulated variable dose trial. Br J Obstet Gynaecol 1989;96(5):607–12.

Holst K, Wilson P. The prevalence of female urinary incontinence and reasons for not seeking treatment. N Z Med J 1988;101:756–8.

Hu T. Impact of urinary incontinence on health-care cost. J Am Geriatr Soc 1990;38:292–5.

Hu T. The cost impact of urinary incontinence on health care services. Paper presented at: National Multi-Specialty Nursing Conference on Urinary Continence; 1994 Jan; Phoenix, AZ.

Hu T, Gabelko K, Weis KA, Fogarty TE, Diokno AC, McCormick KA. Clinical guidelines and cost implications—the case of urinary incontinence. Geriatr Nephrol Urol 1994;4:85–91.

Hu TW, Igou JF, Kaltreider DL, Yu LC, Rohner TJ, Dennis PJ, Craighead WE, Hadley ED, Ory MG. A clinical trial of a behavioral therapy to reduce urinary incontinence in nursing homes. JAMA 1989;261(18):2656–62.

Hu TW, Kaltreider DL, Igou RN. The cost-effectiveness of disposable versus reusable diapers. J Gerontol Nurs 1990;16(2):19–24.

Huland H, Bucher H. Endoscopic bladder neck suspension (Stamey-Pereyra) in female urinary stress incontinence. Eur Urol 1984;10:238–41.

Iosif CS. Sling operation for urinary incontinence. Acta Obstet Gynecol Scand 1985;64:187–90.

Ireton RC, Krieger JN, Cardenas DD, Williams-Burden B, Kelly E, Souci T, Chapman WH. Bladder volume determination using a dedicated, portable ultrasound scanner. J Urol 1990;143(5):909–11.

Jayachandran S, Mooppan UMM, Kim H. Complications from external (condom) urinary drainage devices. Urology 1985 Jan;25(1):31–4.

Jeter KF, Gartley C. Report on public education about incontinence in the United States to the AHCPR urinary incontinence guideline education subcommittee. (Unpublished peer review report.) Spartanburg (SC): Help for Incontinent People, Inc., and Wilmette (IL): The Simon Foundation for Continence; 1994.

Jeter KF, Wagner DB. Incontinence in the American home: a survey of 36,500 people. J Am Geriatr Soc 1990;38:379–83.

Jirovec MM. The impact of daily exercise on the mobility balance and urine control of cognitively impaired nursing home residents. Int J Nurs Stud 1991;28(2):145–51.

Jirovec MM, Wells TJ. Urinary incontinence in nursing home residents with dementia: the mobility-cognition paradigm. Appl Nurs Res 1990 Aug;3(3):112–7.

Johnson DE, Muncie HL, O'Reilly JL, Warren JW. An external urine collection device for incontinent women: evaluation of long-term use. J Am Geriatr Soc 1990;38:1016–22.

Johnson DE, O'Reilly JL, Warren JW. Clinical evaluation of an external urine collection device for nonambulatory incontinent women. J Urol 1989 Mar;141(3):535–7.

Johnson ET. The condom catheter: urinary tract infection and other complications. South Med J 1983 May;76(5):579–82.

Johnson JR, Roberts PL, Olsen RJ, Moyer KA, Stammio E. Prevention of catheter-associated urinary tract infections with silver oxide-coated urinary catheter. J Infect Dis 1990;162:1145–50.

Jones DJ, Shah PJR, Worth PHL. Modified Stamey procedure for bladder neck suspension. Br J Urol 1989;63:157–61.

Joseph C, Jacobson C, Strausbaugh L, Maxwell M, French M, Colling J. Sterile vs clean urinary catheterization. J Am Geriatr Soc 1991;39:1042–6.

Joseph Rowntree Foundation. Evaluating an incontinence helpline. Social Care Research Findings, 17. York, United Kingdom: Joseph Rowntree Foundation; 1991.

Jouppila P, Kauppila A, Ylikorkala O, Ala-Ketola L, Jarvinen PA. Results of operative treatment of stress urinary incontinence with special reference to preoperative clinical and radiological evaluation. Acta Obstet Gynecol Scand 1977;56:409–13.

Judge TG. The use of quinestradol in elderly incontinent women, a preliminary report. Gerontol Clin 1969;11(3):159–64.

Juma S, Little NA, Raz S. Vaginal wall sling: four years later. Urology 1992;34:424–8.

Kadar N. The value of bladder filling in the clinical detection of urine loss and selection of patients for urodynamic testing. Br J Obstet Gynaecol 1988;95(7):698–704.

Kane RL, Garrard J, Skay CL, Radosevich DM. Effects of a geriatric nurse practitioner on process and outcome of nursing home care. Am J Public Health 1989;79(9):1271–7.

Karram MM, Rosenzweig BA, Bhatia NN. Artificial urinary sphincter for recurrent/severe stress incontinence in women. J Reprod Med 1993;38:791–4.

Kaufman M, Lockhart JL, Silverstein MJ, Politano VA. Transurethral polytetrafluoroethylene injection for post-prostatectomy urinary incontinence. J Urol 1984;132:463.

Keating JC, Schulte DC, Miller E. Conservative care of urinary incontinence in the elderly. J Manipulative Physiol Ther 1988;11(4):300–8.

Kersey J. The gauze hammock sling operation in the treatment of stress incontinence. Br J Obstet Gynaecol 1983;90:945.

Kiilholma P, Makinen J. Disappointing effect of endoscopic teflon injection for female stress incontinence. Eur Urol 1991;20:197–9.

Kiilholma P, Makinen J, Chancellor MB, Pitkanen Y, Hirvonen T. Modified Burch colposuspension for stress urinary incontinence in females. Surg Gynecol Obstet 1993;176:111–5.

Kil PJM, Hoekstra JW, van der Meijden APM, Smans AJ, Theeuwes AGM, Schreinemachers LMH. Transvaginal ultrasonography and urodynamic evaluation after suspension operations: comparison among the Gittes, Stamey and Burch suspensions. Am Urol Assoc 1991;146:132–6.

King RB, Carlson CE, Mervine J, Wu Y, Yarkony GM. Clean and sterile intermittent catheterization methods in hospitalized patients with spinal cord injury. Arch Phys Med Rehabil 1992;73:798–802.

Kings Fund. Action on incontinence: report of a working group. Kings Fund Project Paper, no. 43. London: King Edwards Hospital Fund for London; 1983. p. 5–13.

Kirby RS, Whiteway JE. Assessment of the results of Stamey bladder neck suspension. Br J Urol 1989;63:21–3.

Klarskov P, Nielsen KK, Kromman-Andersen B, Maegaard E. Long-term results of pelvic floor training and surgery for female genuine stress incontinence. Int Urogynecol J 1991;2:132–5.

Klein L. Maintenance of healthy skin. J Enterostomal Ther 1988;15(6):227–31.

Klein MC, Gauthier RJ, Robbins JM, Kaczorowski J, Jorgensen SH, Franco ED, Johnson B, Waghorn K, Gelfand MM, Guralnick MS, Luskey GW, Joshi AK. Relationship of episiotomy to perineal trauma and morbidity, sexual dysfunction, and pelvic floor relaxation. Am J Obstet Gynecol 1994;171(3):591–8.

Kockelbergh RC. Clam enterocystoplasty in general urological practice. Br J Urol 1991;68:38–41.

Korda A, Ferry J, Hunter P. Colposuspension for the treatment of female urinary incontinence. Aust N Z J Obstet Gynaecol 1989;29:146.

Korda A, Peat B, Hunter P. Experience with silastic slings for female urinary incontinence. Aust N Z J Obstet Gynaecol 1989;29:150–4.

Kuhan W, Rist M, Zaech GA. Intermittent urethral self catheterization: long-term results. Paraplegia 1991;29:222–32.

Kujansuu E. Urodynamic analysis of successful and failed incontinence surgery. Int J Gynaecol Obstet 1983;21:353–60.

Kumar R, Schreib MH. The changing indications for excretory urography. JAMA 1985;254(3):405–9.

Kunin CM. Blockage of urinary catheters: role of microorganisms and constituents of the urine on formation of encrustations. J Clin Epidemiol 1989;42(9):835–42.

Kunin CM, Chin QF, Chambers S. Indwelling urinary catheters in the elderly. Am J Med 1987a Mar;82:405–11.

Kunin CM, Chin QF, Chambers S. Morbidity and mortality associated with indwelling urinary catheters in elderly patients in a nursing home—confounding due to the presence of associated diseases. J Am Geriatr Soc 1987b;35:1001–6.

Kunin CM, Finkelberg S. Evaluation of an intraurethral lubricating catheter in prevention of catheter-induced urinary tract infections. J Urol 1971 Dec;106:928–30.

Kunkle JC, Payne CK, Whitmore KE. Urinary incontinence: combined biofeedback and electrical stimulation treatment. J Urol Nurs 1993;12(3):537–43.

Kursh ED. Factors influencing the outcome of a no incision endoscopic urethropexy. Surg Gynecol Obstet 1992;175:254–8.

Kursh ED, Angell AH, Resnick MI. Evolution of endoscopic urethropexy: seven year experience with various techniques. Urology 1991;37:428.

Lachs MS, Nachamkin I, Edelstein PH, Goldman J, Feinstein AR, Schwartz JS. Spectrum bias in the evaluation of diagnostic tests: lessons from the rapid dipstick test for urinary tract infection. Ann Intern Med 1992;117:135–40.

Lagace EA, Hansen W, Hickner JM. Prevalence and severity of urinary incontinence in ambulatory adults: an UPR study. J Fam Pract 1993;36(6):610–4.

Lamhut P, Jackson TW, Wall LL. The treatment of urinary incontinence with electrical stimulation in nursing home patients: a pilot study. J Am Geriatr Soc 1992;40:48–52.

Langer R, Ron-El R, Bukovsky I, Caspi E. Colposuspension in patients with combined stress incontinence and detrusor instability. Eur Urol 1988;14:437–9.

Langer R, Ron-El R, Newman M, Herman A, Caspi E. Detrusor instability following colposuspension for urinary stress incontinence. Br J Obstet Gynaecol 1988;95:607–10.

Larson G, Victor A. The frequency-volume chart in genuine stress incontinent women. Neurourol Urodyn 1992;1:23–31.

Leach G, Bavendam T. Prospective evaluation of the Incontan transrectal stimulator in women with urinary incontinence. Neurourol Urodyn 1989;8:231–5.

Leach GE, Raz S. Modified Pereyra bladder neck suspension after previously failed anti-incontinence surgery. Urology 1984;23(4):359–62.

Lehtonen T, Rannikko S, Lindell O, Talja M, Wuokko E, Lindskog M. The effect of phenylpropanolamine on female stress urinary incontinence. Ann Chir Gynaecol 1986;75(4):236–41.

Lekan-Rutledge D, Hogue CC, Miller J. Prompted voiding in the nursing home: effect of clinical and staff management protocols. Gerontologist 1992;32:162.

Lewis RI, Lockhart JL, Politano VA. Periurethral polytetrafluoroethylene injections in incontinent female subjects with neurogenic bladder disease. J Urol 1984;131:459.

Liedberg H, Lundeberg T. Silver alloy coated catheters reduce catheter-associated bacterium. Br J Urol 1990;65:379–81.

Liedberg H, Lundeberg T, Ekman P. Refinements in the coating of urethral catheters reduces the incidence of catheter-associated bacteriuria. Eur Urol 1990;17:236–40.

Light JK, Scott FB. Management of urinary incontinence in women with the artificial urinary sphincter. J Urol 1985;134:476.

Linder A, Leach GE, Raz S. Augmentation cystoplasty in the treatment of neurogenic bladder dysfunction. J Urol 1983;129:491–3.

Lindholm P, Lose G. Terbutaline (Bricanyl) in the treatment of female urge incontinence. Urol Int 1986;41(2):158–60.

Lockhart JL, Ellis GF, Helal M, Pow-Sang JM. Combined cystourethropexy for the treatment of type 3 and complicated female urinary incontinence. J Urol 1990 Apr;143(4):722–5.

Lockhart JL, Maggiolo LF, Politano VA. Modified Burch colposuspension in treatment of female urinary incontinence. Urology 1983;21:382–4.

Lopez Lopez JA, Valdivia Uria JB, Uca Terran A. Percutaneous endoscopic urethro-cervicopexy. Eur Urol 1992;22:167–70.

Lose G, Andersen JI, Kristensen JK. Disposable vaginal surface electrode for urethral sphincter electromyography. Br J Urol 1986;59:408–13.

Lose G, Jorgensen L, Johnsen A. Predictive value of detrusor instability index in surgery for female urinary incontinence. Neurourol Urodyn 1988;7:141–8.

Lose G, Jorgensen L, Thunedborg P. Doxepin in the treatment of female detrusor over-activity: a randomized double-blind crossover study. J Urol 1989 Oct;142(4):1024–6.

Lotenfoe R, O'Kelly JK, Helal M, Lockhart JL. Periurethral polytetrafluoroethylene paste injection in incontinent female subjects: surgical indications and improved surgical technique. J Urol 1993;149:279–82.

Loughlin KR, Whitmore WF, et al. Review of an 8-year experience with modifications of endoscopic suspensions of the bladder neck for female stress urinary incontinence. J Urol 1990;143:44–5.

Low JA. Management of severe anatomic deficiencies of urethral sphincter function by a combined procedure with a fascia lata sling. Am J Obstet Gynecol 1969;105:149.

Lowe DH, Scherz HC, Parsons CL. Urethral pressure profilometry in Scott artificial urinary sphincter. Urology 1988;31:82.

Lucas MG, Thomas DG, Clarke S, Forster DMC. Long-term follow-up of selective sacral neurectomy. Br J Urol 1988;61:218.

Malloy TR, Wein AJ, Carpiniello VL. Surgical success with AMS M800 GU sphincter for male incontinence. Urology 1989;33:274.

Marks JL, Light JK. Management of urinary incontinence after prostatectomy with the artificial urinary sphincter. J Urol 1989;142:302.

McCormick KA, Burgio K. Incontinence: an update on nursing care measures. J Gerontol Nurs 1984;10(10):16–23.

McCormick KA, Burgio LD, Engel BT, Scheve A, Leahy E. Urinary incontinence: an augmented prompted void approach. J Gerontol Nurs 1992 Mar;18(3):3–10.

McCormick KA, Cella M, Scheve A, Engel BT. Cost-effectiveness of treating incontinence in severely mobility-impaired long term care residents. Q Rev Bull 1990;16(12):439–43.

McDowell BJ, Burgio KL, Dombrowski M, Locher JL, Rodriguez E. An interdisciplinary approach to the assessment and behavioral treatment of urinary incontinence in geriatric outpatients. J Am Geriatr Soc 1992;40:370–4.

McDowell BJ, Engberg S, Weber E, Brodak I, Engberg R. Successful treatment using behavioral interventions of urinary incontinence in homebound older adults. Geriatr Nurs 1994;15(6):303–7.

McFall SL, Yerkes AM, Belzer JA, Cowan LD. Urinary incontinence and quality of life in older women: a community demonstration in Oklahoma. Fam Community Health 1994;17(1):64–75.

McGuire EJ. Disorders of the control of bladder contractility. In: Kursh ED, McGuire EJ, editors. Female urology. Philadelphia: Lippincott; 1994. p. 75–82.

McGuire EJ, Appell RA. Transurethral collagen injection for urinary incontinence. Urology 1994;43(4):413–5.

McGuire EJ, Fitzpatrick CC, Wan J, Bloom D, Sandvordenker J, Ritchey M, Gormley EA. Clinical assessment of urethral sphincter function. J Urol 1993;50:1452–4.

McGuire EJ, Letson W, Wang S. Transvaginal urethrolysis after obstructive urethral suspension procedures. J Urol 1989;142:1037–9.

McGuire EJ, Lytton B. Pubovaginal sling procedure for stress incontinence. J Urol 1978;119:82.

McGuire EJ, Savastano JA. Urodynamic findings and clinical status following vesical denervation procedures for control of incontinence. J Urol 1984;132:87.

McGuire EJ, Woodside JR, Borden TA, Weiss RM. Prognostic value of urodynamic testing in myelodysplasia patients. J Urol 1981;126(2):205–9.

McIndoe GA, Jones RW, Grieve BW. The Aldridge sling procedure in the treatment of urinary stress incontinence. Aust N Z Obstet Gynaecol 1987;27:238.

McIntosh LJ, Frahm JD, Mallett VT, Richardson DA. Pelvic floor rehabilitation in the treatment of incontinence. J Reprod Med 1993;38:662–6.

Meyer S, Dhenin T, Schmidt N, DeGrandi P. Subjective and objective effects of intravaginal electrical myostimulation and biofeedback in patients with genuine stress urinary incontinence. Br J Urol 1992;69:584–8.

Meyhoff HH, Gerstenberg TC, Nordling J. Placebo—the drug of choice in female motor urge incontinence? Br J Urol 1983 Feb;55(1):34–7.

Mezey MD, Lynaugh JE, Cartier MN. Nursing homes and nursing care: lessons from the teaching nursing homes. New York: Springer Publishing; 1989.

Middaugh SJ, Whitehead WE, Burgio KL, Engel BT. Biofeedback in treatment of urinary incontinence stroke patients. Biofeedback Self Regul 1989;14(1):44–51.

Milani R, Scalambrino S, Quadri G, Algeri M, Marchesin R. Marshall-Marchetti-Krantz procedure and Burch colposuspension in the surgical treatment of female urinary incontinence. Br J Obstet Gynaecol 1985;92:1050–3.

Milner G, Hills NF. A double-blind assessment of antidepressants in the treatment of 212 enuretic patients. Med J Aust 1968 Jun 1;1(22):943–7.

Mizunaga M, Miyata M, Kaneko S, et al. Intravesical instillation of oxybutynin hydrochloride therapy for patients with neuropathic bladder. Paraplegia 1994;32:25–9.

Mohide EA, Pringle DM, Robertson D, Chambers L. Prevalence of urinary incontinence in patients receiving home care services. Can Med Assoc J 1988;139:953–6.

Mohr DN, Offord KP, Owen RA, Melton LJ. Asymptomatic microhematuria and urologic disease: a population-based study. JAMA 1986;256:224–9.

Moore KH, Hay DM, Imrie AE, Watson A, Goldstein M. Oxybutynin hydrochloride (3 mg) in the treatment of women with idiopathic detrusor instability. Br J Urol 1990 Nov;66(5):479–85.

Moore KH, Richmond DH, Parys BT. Sex distribution of adult idiopathic detrusor instability in relation to childhood bedwetting. Br J Urol 1991;68:479–82.

Moore TF, Saltmarche A. Developing and testing an instrument to assess the information needs of persons with urinary incontinence. Perspectives 1993;17(1):2–6.

Morgan JE. The suprapubic approach to primary stress urinary incontinence. Am J Obstet Gynecol 1973;115:316–20.

Morishita L, Uman GC, Pierson CA. Education on adult urinary incontinence in nursing school curricula: can it be done in two hours? Nurs Outlook 1994;42:123–9.

Morris A, Browne G, Saltmarche A. Urinary incontinence: correlates among cognitively impaired elderly veterans. J Gerontol Nurs 1992;18:33–40.

Morris JN, Hawes C, Murphy K, Nonemaker S. Long term care resident assessment instrument training manual. Baltimore (MD): Health Care Financing Administration; 1990. 279 p.

Motley RC, Barrett DM. Artificial urinary sphincter cuff erosion. Experience with reimplantation in 37 patients. Urology 1990;35:215.

Mouritsen L, Frimodt MC, Moller M. Long-term effect on pelvic floor exercises on female urinary incontinence. Br J Urol 1991;68(1):32–7.

Mouritsen L, Standberg C, Jensen AR, Berget A, Frimodt MC, Folke K. Inter and intra-observer variation of colpo-cysto-urethrography diagnoses. Acta Obstet Gynecol Scand 1993;72(3):2000–4.

Mundy AR. A trial comparing the Stamey bladder neck suspension procedure with colposuspension for the treatment of stress incontinence. Br J Urol 1983;55:687.

Mundy AR, Stephenson TP. "Clam" ileocystoplasty for the treatment of refractory urge incontinence. Br J Urol 1985;57:641.

Murphy WM. Current status of urinary cytology in the evaluation of bladder neoplasms. Hum Pathol 1990;21:886–96.

Nakamura M, Sakurai T, Sugao H, Sonoda T. Maximum electrical stimulation for urge incontinence. Urol Int 1987;42:285–7.

Nakamura M, Sakurai J, Tsujimoto Y, Tada Y. Bladder inhibition by electrical stimulation of the perianal skin. Urol Int 1986;41:62–3.

Narik G, Palmrich AH. A simplified sling operation suitable for routine use. Am J Obstet Gynecol 1962;84:400.

National Center for Health Statistics. The national nursing home survey: 1977 summary for the United States by Van Nostrand JF, et al. (DHEW Publication No. 79-1794). Vital and health statistics. Series 13, No. 43. Washington (DC): Health Resources Services Administration, U.S. Government Printing Office, 1979.

National Institutes of Health. Urinary Incontinence in Adults. National Institutes of Health Consensus Development Conference. J Am Geriatr Soc 1990;38:265–72.

National Kidney and Urologic Diseases Advisory Board. Barriers to rehabilitation of persons with end-stage renal disease or chronic urinary incontinence. Workshop summary report; 1994 Mar 7–9; Bethesda, MD.

Netto NR, Lemos GC, Palma PCR, Fiuza JL. Comparison of the Stamey bladder neck suspension procedure with a modified endoscopic suspension for the treatment of stress urinary incontinence. Eur Urol 1988;15:62–5.

Nielsen E, Lundvall F. Urethrovaginal fixation to Cooper's ligament (Burch) in the treatment of incontinence. Acta Chir Scand Suppl 1973;433:118–20.

Nitti VW, Bregg KJ, Sussman EM, Raz S. The Raz bladder neck suspension in patients 65 years and older. J Urol 1993;149:802–7.

Nitti VW, Raz S. Obstruction following anti-incontinence procedures: diagnosis and treatment with transvaginal urethrolysis. J Urol 1994 Jul;152(1):93–8.

Noelker L. Incontinence in elderly cared for by family. Gerontologist 1987;27:194–200.

Nordling J, Holm-Bentzen M, Hald T. The AMS artificial urinary sphincter on the bulbous urethra. Scand J Urol Nephrol 1986;20:165.

Nordling J, Steven K, Meyhoff HH, Hald T. Subtrigonal phenol injection: lack of effect in the treatment of detrusor hyperactivity. Neurourol Urodyn 1986;5:449.

Norton PA, MacDonald LD, Sedgwick PM, Stanton SL. Distress and delay associated with urinary incontinence, frequency, and urgency in women. BMJ 1988 Nov 5;29:1187–9.

Norton P, Peattie A, Stanton S. Estimation of urinary residual by palpation. Neurourol Urodyn 1989;8(4):330–1.

Nygaard IE, Thompson FL, Svengalis SL, Albright JP. Urinary incontinence in elite nulliparous athletes. Obstet Gynecol 1994;84(2):183–7.

O'Brien J, Austin M, Sethi P, O'Boyle P. Urinary incontinence: prevalence, need for treatment, and effectiveness of intervention by nurse. BMJ 1991 Nov 23;303:1308–12.

O'Connell HE, McGuire EJ, Aboseif S, Usui A. Transurethral collagen therapy in women. J Urol. In press.

O'Donnell P, Doyle R. Biofeedback therapy technique for treatment of urinary incontinence. Urology 1991;37:432–6.

O'Donnell PD, Beck C, Walls RC. Serial incontinence assessment in elderly inpatient men. J Rehab Res Dev 1990;27(1):1–9.

Ogundipe A, Rosenzweig BA. Modified suburethral sling procedure for treatment of recurrent or severe stress urinary incontinence. Surg Gynecol Obstet 1992;175:173–6.

Ohlsson BL, Fall M, Frankenberg-Sommar S. Effects of external and direct pudendal nerve maximal electrical stimulation in the treatment of the uninhibited overactive bladder. Br J Urol 1989;64:374–80.

Olah KS, Bridges N, Denning J, Farrar DJ. The conservative management of patients with symptoms of stress incontinence: a randomized, prospective study comparing weighted vaginal cones and interferential therapy. Am J Obstet Gynecol 1990;162(1):87–92.

Opsomer RJ, Klarskov P, Holm-Bentzen M, Hald T. Long-term results of superselective sacral nerve resection for motor urge incontinence. Scand J Urol Nephrol 1984;18:101.

Osther PJ, Rohl HF. Teflon injections in post-prostatectomy incontinence. Scand J Urol Nephrol 1988;22:171–4.

Ouslander J, Kane R, Abrass I. Urinary incontinence in elderly nursing home patients. JAMA 1982;248:1194–8.

Ouslander JG. Asymptomatic bacteriuria and incontinence [letter]. J Am Geriatr Soc 1989;37(2):197–8.

Ouslander JG, Bruskewitz R. Disorders of micturition in the aging patient. Adv Int Med 1989;34:165–90.

Ouslander JG, Greengold B, Chen S. Complications of chronic indwelling urinary catheters among male nursing home patients: a prospective study. J Urol 1987a Nov;138:1191–5.

Ouslander JG, Greengold B, Chen S. External catheter use and urinary tract infections among incontinent male nursing home patients. J Am Geriatr Soc 1987b Dec;35:1063–70.

Ouslander JG, Hepps K, Raz S, Su HL. Genitourinary dysfunction in a geriatric outpatient population. J Am Geriatr Soc 1986;34(7):507–14.

Ouslander JG, Leach GE, Staskin DR. Simplified tests of lower urinary tract function in evaluation of geriatric urinary incontinence. J Am Geriatr Soc 1989;37(8):706–14.

Ouslander JG, Leach G, Staskin D, Abelson S, Blaustein J, Morishita L, Raz S. Prospective evaluation of assessment strategy for geriatric urinary incontinence. J Amer Geriatr Soc 1989;37(8):715–24.

Ouslander JG, Palmer MH, Rovner BW, German PS. Urinary incontinence in nursing homes: incidence remission and associated factors. J Am Geriatr Soc 1993;41(10):1083–9.

Ouslander J, Schnelle J, Simmons S, Bates-Jenson B, Zeitlin M. The dark side of incontinence in nursing home residents. J Am Geriatr Soc 1993;41:371–6.

Ouslander JG, Schnelle J, Uman GC, Fingold S, Glater Nigam J, Tuico E, Bates-Jensen B. Predictors of successful prompted voiding among incontinent nursing home residents. JAMA 1995;273:1366–70.

Ouslander JG, Simmons S, Tuico E, Nigam JG, Fingold S, Bates-Jensen B, Schnelle JF. Use of a portable ultrasound device to measure post-void residual volume among incontinent nursing home residents. J Am Geriatr Soc 1994;42(11):1189–92.

Ouslander JG, Zarit SH, Orr NK, Muira SA. Incontinence among elderly community-dwelling dementia patients: characteristics, management, and impact on caregivers. J Am Geriatr Soc 1990;38:440–5.

Palmer JH, Worth PHL, Exton-Smith AN. Flunarizine: a once daily therapy for urinary incontinence. Lancet 1981;2:279–81.

Palmer MH. A health promotion perspective of urinary continence. Nurs Outlook 1994 Jul/Aug;42(4):163–9.

Palmer MH. Nurses' knowledge and beliefs about continence interventions in long-term care. J Adv Nurs 1995;21:1065–72.

Palmer MH, Bennett RG, Marks J, McCormick KA, Engel BT. Urinary incontinence: a program that works. J Long Term Care Admin 1994;22(2):19–25.

Palmer MH, German PS, Ouslander JG. Risk factors for urinary incontinence one year after nursing home admission. Res Nurs Health 1991;14:405–12.

Palmer MH, McCormick KA, Langford A, Langlois J, Alvaran M. Continence outcomes: documentation on medical records in the nursing home environment. J Nurs Care Qual 1992;6(3):36–43.

Panel for the Prediction and Prevention of Pressure Ulcers in Adults. Pressure ulcers in adults: prediction and prevention. Clinical practice guideline, no. 3. AHCPR Publication No. 92-0047. Rockville (MD): U.S. Department of Health and Human Services. Public Health Service, Agency for Health Care Policy and Research; May 1992.

Park GS, Miller EJ Jr. Surgical treatment of stress urinary incontinence: a comparison of the Kelly plication, Marshall-Marchetti-Krantz, and Pereyra procedures. Obstet Gynecol 1988;71:575–9.

Parra RO, Shaker L. Experience with a simplified technique for the treatment of female stress urinary incontinence. Br J Urol 1990;66:615–7.

Parulkar BG, Barrett DM. Application of the A-800 artificial sphincter for intractable urinary incontinence in females. Surg Gynecol Obstet 1990;171:131.

Pearson B, Droessler D. Continence through nursing care. Geriatr Nurs 1988;9(6):347–9.

Peattie AB, Plevnik S. Cones versus physiotherapy as conservative management of genuine stress incontinence. Neurourol Urodyn 1988;7(3):72–3.

Peattie AB, Plevnik S, Stanton SL. Vaginal cones: a conservative method of treating genuine stress incontinence. Br J Obstet Gynaecol 1988;95:1049–53.

Pengelly AW, Booth CM. A prospective trial of bladder training as treatment for detrusor instability. Br J Urol 1980;52:463–6.

Penttinen J, Kaar K, Kauppila A. Colposuspension and transvaginal bladder neck suspension in the treatment of stress incontinence. Gynecol Obstet Invest 1989;28:101–5.

Penttinen J, Lindholm EL, Kaar K, Kauppila A. Successful colposuspension in stress urinary incontinence reduces bladder neck mobility and increases pressure transmission to the urethra. Arch Gynecol Obstet 1989;244:233–8.

Pereyra AJ, Lebherz TB, Growdon WA, Powers JA. Pubourethral supports in perspective: modified Pereyra procedure for urinary incontinence. Obstet Gynecol 1982;59:643.

Perkash I, Giroux J. Clean intermittent catheterization in spinal cord injury patients: a follow-up study. J Urol 1993 May;149:1068–71.

Pieper B, Cleland V. An external urine-collection device for women: a clinical trial. J ET Nurs 1993;20:51–5.

Pieper B, Cleland V, Johnson DE, O'Reilly JL. Inventing urine incontinence devices for women. Image J Nurs Sch 1989 Winter;21(4):205–9.

Plevnik S, Joney J, Vrtacnik P, et al. Short term electrical simulation: home treatment for urinary incontinence. World J Urol 1986;4:24–6.

Politano VA. Transurethral polytef injection for post-prostatectomy urinary incontinence. Br J Urol 1992;69:26–8.

Pope AJ, Shaw PJR, Coptcoat MH, Worth PHL. Changes in bladder function following a surgical alteration in outflow resistance. Neurourol Urodyn 1990;9:503–8.

Pow-Sang JM, Lockhart JL, Suarez A, Lansman H, Politano VA. Female urinary incontinence: preoperative selection, surgical complications and results. J Urol 1986;136:831–3.

Quinn MJ, Beynon J, Mortensen NJM, Smith PJB. Transvaginal endosonography: a new method to study the anatomy of the lower urinary tract in urinary stress incontinence. Br J Urol 1988;62(5):414–8.

Ramon F, Mekras JA, Webster GD. The outcome of transvaginal cysturethropexy in patients with anatomical stress urinary incontinence and outlet weakness. J Urol 1990;144:106–9.

Raz S. Modified bladder neck suspension for female stress incontinence. Urology 1981;17:82–5.

Raz S, Ehrlich RM, Zeidman EJ, Alarcon A, McLaughlin S. Surgical treatment of the incontinent female patient with myelomeningocele. J Urol 1988;139:524.

Raz S, Sussman EM, Erickson DB, Bregg KJ, Nitti VW. The Raz bladder neck suspension: results in 206 patients. J Urol 1992;148:845–50.

Resnick NM. Voiding dysfunction in the elderly. In: Yalla SV, McGuire EJ, Elbadawi A, Blaivas JG, eds. Neurourology and urodynamics: principles and practice. New York: Macmillan, 1988; 303–30.

Resnick NM, Baumann MM. A national assessment strategy for urinary incontinence in nursing homes. Neurourol Urodyn 1990;9:411–3.

Resnick NM, Yalla SV. Management of urinary incontinence in the elderly. N Engl J Med 1985;313:800–5.

Resnick NM, Yalla SV, Laurino E. The pathophysiology of urinary incontinence among institutionalized elderly persons. N Engl J Med 1989;320(1):1–7.

Richardson DA, Ramahi A, Chalas E. Surgical management of stress incontinence in patients with low urethral pressure. Gynecol Obstet Invest 1991;131:106–9.

Richmond DH, Sutherst JR. Burch colposuspension or sling for stress incontinence? A prospective study using transrectal ultrasound. Br J Urol 1989a;64:600–3.

Richmond DH, Sutherst JR. Clinical application of transrectal ultrasound for the investigation of the incontinent patient. Br J Urol 1989b;63(6):605–9.

Ridley JH. Appraisal of the Goeb ell-Frangenheim-Stoeckel sling procedure. Am J Obstet Gynecol 1966;95:714.

Rife CC, Farrow GM, Utz DC. Urine cytology of transitional cell neoplasms. Urol Clin North Am 1979;6:599–612.

Riva D, Casolati E. Oxybutynin chloride in the treatment of female idiopathic bladder instability. Clin Exp Obstet Gynecol 1984;11(1–2):37–42.

Robertson AS, Davies JB, Webb RJ, Neal DE. Bladder augmentation and replacement. Urodynamic and clinical review of 25 patients. Br J Urol 1991;68:590–7.

Robinson JM, Brocklehurst JC. Emepronium bromide and flavoxate hydrochloride in the treatment of urinary incontinence associated with detrusor instability in elderly women. Br J Urol 1983 Aug;55(4):371–6.

Rockswald GL, Chou SN, Bradley WE. Re-evaluation of differential sacral rhizotomy for neurological bladder disease. J Neurosurg 1978;48:773.

Rose M, Baigis-Smith J, Smith D, Newman D. Behavioral management of urinary incontinence in homebound older adults. Home Healthcare Nurse 1990;8:10–5.

Rosenbaum TP, Shaw PJR, Worth PHL. Trans-trigonal phenol failed the test of time. Br J Urol 1990;66:164.

Rubin M, Berger SA, Zodda FN Jr, Guenwald R. Effect of catheter replacement on bacterial counts in urine aspirated from indwelling catheters. J Infect Dis 1980 Aug;142:291.

Ruther M, Helbing C. Health care financing trends: use and cost of home health services under Medicare. Health Care Financing Rev 1988;10:105–8.

Ruwaldt MM. Irrigation of indwelling urinary catheters. Urology 1983 Feb;21:127–9.

Samsioe G, Jansson I, Mellstrom D, Svanborg A. Occurrence, nature and treatment of urinary incontinence in a 70-year-old female population. Maturitas 1985 Nov;7(4):335–42.

Sand PK, Bowen LW, Ostergard DR, Nakanishi AM. Hysterectomy and prior incontinence surgery as risk factors for failed retropubic cystourethropexy. J Reprod Med 1988;33:171–4.

Sand PK, Brubaker LT, Novak T. Standing incremental cystometry as a screening method for detrusor instability. Obstet Gynecol 1991;77:453–7.

Sand PK, Richardson DA, Staskin DR, Swift SE, Appell RA, Whitmore KE, Ostergard DR. Pelvic floor electrical stimulation in the treatment of genuine stress incontinence: a multicenter, placebo-controlled trial. Am J Obstet Gynecol 1995;173:72–9.

Santarosa RP, Blaivas JG. Periurethral injection of autologous fat for the treatment of sphincteric incompetence. J Urol 1994;151:607–11.

Scheve A, Engel B, McCormick K, Leahy E. Exercise in continence. Geriatr Nurs 1991 May/June;12(3):124.

Schnelle JF. Treatment of urinary incontinence in nursing home patients by prompted voiding. J Am Geriatr Soc 1990;38:356–60.

Schnelle JF, Newman DR, Fogarty T. Management of patient continence in long-term care nursing facilities. Gerontologist 1990;30:373–6.

Schnelle JF, Newman DR, Fogarty TE, Wallston D, Ory M. Assessment and quality control of incontinence care in long term nursing facilities. J Am Geriatr Soc 1991;39(2):165–71.

Schnelle JF, Newman DR, White M, Abbey J, Wallston KA, Fogarty T, Ory MG. Maintaining continence in NH residents through the application of industrial quality control. Gerontologist 1993;33:114–21.

Schnelle JF, Sowell VA, Hu TW, Traughber B. Reduction of urinary incontinence in nursing homes: does it reduce or increase costs? J Am Geriatr Soc 1988;36:34–9.

Schreiter F. Bulbar artificial sphincter. Eur Urol 1985;11:294.

Schrier RW. Body fluid volume regulation in health and disease. Ann Intern Med 1990;113(2):155.

Schulman CC, Simon J, Wespes E, Germeau F. Endoscopic injection of Teflon for female urinary incontinence. Eur Urol 1983;9:246.

Schwartz MS. Biofeedback: practitioner's guide. New York: Guilford Press; 1995.

Scotti RF, Ostergard DR. Predictive vale of urethroscopy in genuine stress incontinence and vesical instability. Int Urogynecol J 1993;4(5):255–8.

Sethia KK, Webb RJ, Neal DE. Urodynamic study of ileocystoplasty in the treatment of idiopathic detrusor instability. Br J Urol 1991;67:286–90.

Shah PJR, Holder PD. Comparison of Stamey and Pereyra-Raz bladder neck suspensions. Br J Urol 1989;64:481–4.

Shull BL, Baden WF. A six-year experience with paravaginal defect repair for stress urinary incontinence. Am J Obstet Gynecol 1989;160:1432–40.

Shumaker SA, Wyman JF, Uebersax JS, McClish D, Fantl JA. Health-related quality-of-life measures for women with urinary incontinence—the incontinence impact questionnaire and the urogenital distress inventory. Qual Life Res 1994;3(5):291–306.

Sidi AA, Becher EF, Reddy PK, Dykstra DD. Augmentation enterocystoplasty for the management of voiding dysfunction in spinal cord injury patients. J Urol 1990;143:83.

Siu AL, Beers MH, Morgenstern H. The geriatric "medical and public health" imperative revisited. J Am Geriatr Soc 1993;41:78–84.

Skelly J, Flint AJ. Urinary incontinence associated with dementia. J Am Geriatr Soc 1995;43:286–94.

Smart RF. Polytef paste for urinary incontinence. Aust N Z J Surg 1991;61:663–6.

Smyer M, Brannon D, Cohn M. Improving nursing home care through training and job redesign. Gerontologist 1992;32(3):327–33.

Sogbein SK, Awad SA. Behavioral treatment of urinary incontinence in geriatric patients. Can Med Assoc J 1982;127:863–4.

Sowell VA, Schnelle JF, Hu TW, Traughber B. A cost comparison of five methods of managing urinary incontinence. Q Rev Biol 1987 Dec;411–4.

Special Committee on Aging, United States Senate. Developments in aging: 1987, vol. 3. The long-term care challenge (Dept. 100-291). Washington (DC): US Government Printing Office; 1988.

Spencer JR, O'Conor VJ, Schaeffer AJ. A comparison of endoscopic suspension of the vesical neck with suprapubic vesicourethropexy for treatment of stress urinary incontinence. J Urol 1987;137:411–5.

Stamey TA. Endoscopic suspension of the vesical neck for urinary incontinence in females. Ann Surg 1980;192:465.

Stanisic TH, Jennings CE, Miller JI. Polytetrafluoroethylene injection for post-prostatectomy incontinence: experience with 20 patients during 3 years. J Urol 1991;146:1575–7.

Stanton SL, Cardozo LD. Results of the colposuspension operation for incontinence and prolapse. Br J Obstet Gynaecol 1979;86:693–7.

Stanton SL, Hilton P, Norton C, Cardozo, L. Clinical and urodynamic effects of anterior colporrhaphy and vaginal hysterectomy for prolapse with and without incontinence. Br J Obstet Gynaecol 1982;89:459–60.

Stanton SL, Williams JE, Ritchie D. The colposuspension operation for urinary incontinence. Br J Obstet Gynaecol 1976;83:890–5.

Starer P, Lobow LS. Obscuring urinary continence: diapering of the elderly. J Am Geriatr Soc 1985;113(12):842–6.

Staskin DR, Zimmern PE, Hadley HR, Raz S. The pathophysiology of stress incontinence. Urol Clin N Am 1985;12:271–8.

Steel SS, Cox C, Stanton SL. Long-term follow-up of detrusor instability following the colposuspension operation. Br J Urol 1985;58:138–42.

Stoddart G. Research project into the effect of pelvic exercises on genuine stress incontinence. Physiotherapy 1983;69(5):148–9.

Stower MJ, Massey JA, Feneley RC. Urethral closure in management of urinary incontinence. Urology 1989 Nov;34(5):246–8.

Strahan GW. An overview of home health and hospice care patients: preliminary data from the 1993 National Home and Hospice Care Survey. Advance data from Vital and Health Statistics; No. 256. Hyattsville (MD): National Center for Health Statistics; 1994.

Strawbridge LR, Kramer SA, Castillo OA, Barrett DM. Augmentation cystoplasty and the artificial genitourinary sphincter. J Urol 1989;142:297.

Stricker P, Haylen B. Injectable collagen for type 3 female stress incontinence: the first 50 Australian patients. Med J Aust 1993;158:89–91.

Susset JG, Galea G, Read L. Biofeedback therapy for female incontinence due to low urethral resistance. J Urol 1990 Jun;143(6):1205–8.

Sutherst JR, Brown MC. Comparison of single and multichannel cystometry in diagnosing bladder instability. BMJ 1984;288:1720–3.

Tapp AJ, Cardozo LD, Versi E, Cooper D. The treatment of detrusor instability in postmenopausal women with oxybutynin chloride: a double-blind placebo controlled study. Br J Obstet Gynaecol 1990 Jun;97(6):521–6.

Taylor MC, Bates CP. A double-blind crossover trial of baclofen: a new treatment for the unstable bladder syndrome. Br J Urol 1979 Dec;51(6):504–5.

Tenney JH, Warren JW. Bacteriuria in women with long-term indwelling catheters: paired comparison of the indwelling and replacement catheter. J Infect Dis 1988;157:199–202.

Terpenning MS, Allada R, Kauffman CA. Intermittent urethral catheterization in the elderly. J Am Geriatr Soc 1989 May;37:411–6.

Thomas TM, Plymat KR, Blannin J, Meade TW. Prevalence of urinary incontinence. BMJ 1980;281:1243–5.

Thompson RL, Haley CE, Searcy MA, Guenthner SM, Kaiser DL, Groschel HM, et al. Catheter-associated bacteriuria. JAMA 1984;251(6):747–51.

Thunedborg P, Fischer-Rasmussen W, Jensen SB. Stress urinary incontinence and posterior bladder suspension defects: results of vaginal repair versus Burch colposuspension. Acta Obstet Gynecol Scand 1990;69:55–9.

Thuroff JW, Bunke B, Ebner A, Faber P, de Geeter P, Hannappel J, Heidler H, Madersbacher H, Melchior H, Schafer W. Randomized, double-blind, multicenter trial on treatment of frequency, urgency and incontinence related to detrusor hyperactivity: oxybutynin versus propantheline versus placebo. J Urol 1991;145(4):813–7.

Topper JR, Holliday PJ, Fernie GR. Bladder volume estimation in the elderly using a portable ultrasound-based measurement device. J Med Eng Technol 1993 May;17(3):99–103.

Torring J, Petersen T, Kelmar B, Sogaard I. Selective sacral rootlet neurectomy in the treatment of detrusor hyperreflexia. J Neurosurg 1988;68:241.

Uebersax JS, Wyman JF, Shumaker SA, McClish DK, Fantl JA, Continence Program for Women Research Group. Short forms to assess life quality and symptom distress for urinary incontinence in women: the incontinence impact questionnaire and the urogenital distress inventory. Neurourol Urodyn 1995;14:131–9.

US Department of Health and Human Services, Public Health Service. Healthy People 2000. National Health Promotion and Disease Prevention Objectives. DHHS Publication No. (PHS) 91-50212. Washington (DC): US Government Printing Office; 1990.

Utz DC, Zincke H. The masquerade of bladder cancer in situ as interstitial cystitis. J Urol 1974;111:160–1.

Van Geelen M, Theeuwes AGM, Eskes TKAB, Martin CB. The clinical and urodynamic effects of anterior vaginal repair and Burch colposuspensoin. Am J Obstet Gynecol 1988;159:137–44.

Varner RE. Retropubic long-needle suspension procedures for stress urinary incontinence. Am J Obstet Gynecol 1990;164:551–7.

Vehkalahti I, Kivela SL, Seppanen J. Are cystometric and cystoscopic examinations of any value for disabled incontinent elderly? Scand J Prim Health Care 1986;4:243–7.

Vesey SG, Rivett A, O'Boyle PJ. Teflon injection in female subjects incontinence. Effect on urethral pressure profile and flow rate. Br J Urol 1988;62:39.

Vodusek DB, Plevnik S, Vrtacnik P, Janez J. Detrusor inhibition on selective pudendal nerve stimulation in the perineum. Neurourol Urodyn 1988;6:389–93.

Vordermark JS, Brannen GE, Wettlauffer JN, Modarelli RO. Suprapubic endoscopic vesical neck suspension. J Urol 1979;122:165–7.

Wagner A, Colling J. Resistance to change: understanding the aides' point of view. J Long Term Care Admin 1993;21(2):27–30.

Wahlquist GI, McGuire E, Greene W, Herlihy E. Intermittent catheterization and urinary tract infection. Rehabil Nurs 1983 Jan-Feb;8(1):18–9, 41.

Walker GT, Texter JH. Success and patient satisfaction following the Stamey procedure for stress urinary incontinence. J Urol 1992;147:1521–3.

Wall LL, Stanton SL. Transvesical phenol injection of pelvic nerve plexuses in females with refractory urge incontinence. Br J Urol 1989;63:465.

Walter S, Kjaergaard B, Lose G, Andersen JT, Heisterberg L, Jakobsen H, Klarskov P, Moller-Hansen K, Lindskog M. Stress urinary incontinence in postmenopausal women treated with oral estrogen (estriol) and an alpha-adrenoceptor-stimulating agent (phenylpropanolamine): a randomized double-blind placebo-controlled study. Int Urogynecol J 1990;1(2):74–9.

Wan J, McGuire EJ, Bloom DA, Ritchey ML. Stress leak point pressure: a diagnostic tool for incontinent children. J Urol 1993;150:700–2.

Wang Y, Hadley HR. Management of persistent or recurrent urinary incontinence after placement of artificial urinary sphincter. J Urol 1991;146:1005–6.

Warren JW. Urine-collection devices for use in adults with urinary incontinence. J Am Geriatr Soc 1990;38:364–7.

Warren JW, Muncie HL, Hall-Craggs M. Acute pyelonephritis associated with bacteriuria during long-term catheterization: a prospective clinicopathological study. J Infect Dis 1988 Dec;158(6):1341–6.

Warren JW, Steinberg L, Hebel JR, Tenney JH. The prevalence of urethral catheterization in Maryland nursing homes. Arch Intern Med 1989 July;149:1535–7.

Warwick DJ, Abrams P. The perineal artificial sphincter for acquired incontinence: a cut and dried solution? Br J Urol 1990;66:495–9.

Webb RJ, Lawson AL, Neal DE. Clean intermittent self-catheterization in 172 adults. Br J Urol 1990;65:2023.

Webster GD, Perez LM, Khoury JM, Timmons SL. Management of type II stress urinary incontinence using artificial urinary sphincter. Urology 1992;39:499–503.

Wein AJ. Pharmacologic treatment of incontinence. J Am Geriatr Soc 1990;38(3):317–25.

Wells T, Brink C, Diokno A, Wolfe R, Gillis G. Pelvic muscle exercise for stress urinary incontinence in elderly women. J Am Geriatr Soc 1991;39:785–91.

Wheelahan J. Long-term results of colposuspension. Br J Urol 1990;65:329–32.

Williams ME, Gaylord SA. Role of functional assessment in the evaluation of urinary incontinence: National Institutes of Health Consensus Development Conference on Urinary Incontinence in Adults, Bethesda, MD, October 3–5, 1988. J Am Geriatr Soc 1990;38(3):296–9.

Williams ME, Pannill FC III. Urinary incontinence in the elderly: pathophysiology, diagnosis and treatment. Ann Intern Med 1982;97(6):895–907.

Wilson PD. Conservative management of urethral sphincter incompetence. Clin Obstet Gynecol 1990;33:330–45.

Wilson PD, Borland M. Vaginal cones for the treatment of genuine stress incontinence. Aust N Z J Obstet Gynaecol 1990;30:157–60.

Wilson PD, Faragher B, Butler B, Bullock D, Robinson EL, Brown AD. Treatment with oral piperazine oestrone sulphate for genuine stress incontinence in postmenopausal women. Br J Obstet Gynaecol 1987 Jun;94(6):568–74.

Wujanto R, O'Reilley PH. Stamey needle suspension for stress urinary incontinence. Br J Urol 1989;63:162–4.

Wyman J, Elswick RK Jr, Ory MG, Wilson MS, Fantl JA. Influence of functional, urological, and environmental characteristics on urinary incontinence in community-dwelling older women. Nurs Res 1993;42(5):270–5.

Wyman JF, Choi SC, Harkins SW, Wilson MS, Fantl JA. The urinary diary in evaluation of urinary incontinence in women: a test retest analysis. Obstet Gynecol 1988;71(6 pt. 1):812–7.

Wyndaele J, Maes D. Clean intermittent self-catheterization: a 12-year follow-up. J Urol 1990 May;143:906–8.

Zeegers AGM, Kiesswetter H, Kramer AEJL, Jonas U. Conservative therapy of frequency, urgency and urge incontinence: a double-blind clinical trial of flavoxate hydrochloride, oxybutynin chloride, emepronium bromide and placebo. World J Urol 1987;5(1):57–61.

Zimmern PE, Hadley HR, Leach GE, Raz S. Female urethral obstruction after Marshall-Marchetti-Krantz operation. J Urol 1987;138:517–20.

Zollner-Nielsen M, Samuelsson SM. Maximal electrical stimulation of patients with frequency, urgency, and urge incontinence. Report of 38 cases. Acta Obstet Gynecol Scand 1992;71(8):629–31.

Zorzitto ML, Holliday PJ, Jewett MAS, Herschorn S, Fernie GR. Oxybutynin chloride for geriatric urinary dysfunction: a double-blind placebo-controlled study. Age Ageing 1989 May;18(3):195–200.

Zorzitto ML, Jewett MAS, Fernie GR, Holliday PJ, Bartlett S. Effectiveness of propantheline bromide in the treatment of geriatric patients with detrusor instability. Neurourol Urodyn 1986;5(2):133–40.

Abbreviations

ADL	Activities of Daily Living
BPH	Benign prostatic hyperplasia
BUN	Blood urea nitrogen
CMG	Cystometrogram
DHIC	Detrusor hyperactivity with impaired bladder contractility
DI	Detrusor instability
EMG	Electromyography
HCFA	Health Care Financing Administration
ISD	Intrinsic sphincter deficiency
MDS	Minimum Data Set
MMSE	Mini Mental State Examination
NSAID	Nonsteroidal anti-inflammatory drug
PME	Pelvic muscle exercise
PPA	Phenylpropanolamine
PVR	Postvoid residual volume
RAI	Resident Assessment Instrument
RAP	Resident Assessment Protocol
SUI	Stress urinary incontinence
TCA	Tricyclic antidepressant
UI	Urinary incontinence
UPP	Urethral pressure profilmetry
UTI	Urinary tract infection

Glossary

Absorbent products. Pads and garments, either disposable or reusable, worn to contain urinary incontinence or uncontrolled urine leakage. Absorbent products include shields, guards, undergarment pads, combination pad-pant systems, diaperlike garments, and bed pads.

Algorithm. A step-by-step method for solving a problem. In health care decisionmaking, an algorithm is a defined and prescribed sequential process whereby clinical and diagnostic findings at a particular point in the process determine the next diagnostic, clinical, or therapeutic decision or action to be made or taken.

Anti-incontinence surgery. The use of surgical procedures to treat urinary incontinence (see artificial urinary sphincter, bladder suspension, periurethral bulking injections, sling procedures).

Artificial urinary sphincter. A mechanical device surgically implanted into the patient that consists of a cuff, placed around the bulbar urethra or bladder neck, a pressure-regulating balloon, and a pump. The device is used to control opening and closing of the urethra manually and is the most commonly used surgical procedure for the treatment of male urethral insufficiency.

Behavioral techniques. Specific interventions designed to alter the relationship between the patient's symptoms and his/her behavior and/or environment for the treatment of maladaptive urinary voiding patterns. This may be achieved by modification of the behavior and/or environment of the patient (see biofeedback, bladder training, electrical stimulation, habit training, pelvic muscle exercises, prompted voiding).

Benign prostatic hyperplasia (BPH). A common disorder of men over the age of 50 characterized by enlargement of the prostate which may press against the urethra and obstruct the flow of urine. BPH is the most common cause of such anatomic obstruction in elderly men.

Biofeedback. A behavioral technique by which information about a normally unconscious physiologic process is presented to the patient and the clinician as a visual, auditory, or tactile signal. The signal is derived from a measurable physiologic parameter which is subsequently used in an educational process to accomplish a specific therapeutic result. The signal is displayed in a quantitative way, and the patient is taught how to alter it and thus control the physiologic process.

Bladder suspension. Also called bladder neck suspension. A term for several surgical procedures employed to treat urethral hypermobility by elevating and securing the bladder to its proper position within the body. The two major types of bladder suspension surgical procedures are:

Retropubic suspension. Consists of several different surgical techniques performed through a low abdominal incision. All techniques are designed to elevate the lower urinary tract within the retropubic space, differing only in the structures used to achieve the elevation.

Needle bladder neck suspension. Consists of several different surgical techniques performed through a vaginal approach and small low abdominal incision; all involve the use of a long needle to transfer the sutures adjacent to the urethra and bladder neck through the retropubic space into the abdominal wall anterior to the rectus fascia where the sutures are fastened or anchored.

Bladder training. A behavioral technique that requires the patient to resist or inhibit the sensation of urgency (the strong desire to urinate), to postpone voiding, and to urinate according to a timetable rather than to the urge to void.

Catheterization. Techniques for managing urinary incontinence that involve the use of a slender tube inserted through the urethra or through the anterior abdominal wall into the bladder, urinary reservoir, or urinary conduit to allow urine drainage (see indwelling catheters, intermittent catheterization).

Clinical practice guideline. A set of systematically developed statements or recommendations designed to assist practitioner and patient decisions about appropriate health care for specific clinical circumstances. Such guidelines are designed to assist health care practitioners in the prevention, diagnosis, treatment, and management of specific clinical conditions.

Condom catheters. A condomlike device placed over the penis to allow bladder drainage and collection of urine (see external (condom) catheters).

Cystometry. A test used to assess the function of the bladder by measuring the pressure/volume relationship of the bladder. Cystometry is used to assess detrusor activity, sensation, capacity, and compliance. There are different variations of the test depending on the problem being investigated, but regardless of the technique, cystometry involves insertion of a catheter into the bladder.

Cystourethrography. The use of x-ray imaging to examine the urinary bladder and urethra. In voiding cystourethrography, an x-ray picture of the bladder and urethra is obtained during urination.

Cystoscopy. Also called "cystourethroscopy." A procedure used to diagnose urinary tract disorders and provide a direct view of the urethra and bladder by inserting a flexible scope into the urethra and then into the bladder.

Decreased bladder compliance. A failure to store urine in the bladder caused by the loss of bladder wall elasticity and of bladder accommodation. This condition may result from radiation cystitis or from inflammatory bladder conditions such as chemical cystitis, interstitial cystitis, and certain neurologic bladder disorders.

Detrusor. General term for any part of the body that pushes down. In the urinary system, the detrusor muscle is the smooth muscle in the wall of the urinary bladder that contracts the bladder and expels the urine.

Detrusor sphincter dyssynergia (DSD). An inappropriate contraction of the external sphincter concurrent with an involuntary contraction of the detrusor. In the adult, DSD is a common feature of neurologic voiding disorders.

Detrusor hyperactivity with impaired bladder contractility (DHIC). A condition characterized by involuntary detrusor contractions in which patients either are unable to empty their bladder completely or can empty their bladder completely only with straining due to poor contractility of the detrusor.

Detrusor instability (unstable bladder). Involuntary detrusor contraction in the absence of associated neurologic disorders (see urge incontinence).

Electrical stimulation. The application of electric current to stimulate or inhibit the pelvic viscera or their nerve supply in order to induce a direct therapeutic response.

Electromyography (EMG). The study of electrical potentials generated by the depolarization of muscle. EMG of the striated urethral sphincter measures the integrity and function of its nerves and is used to evaluate the neurophysiologic status of the urinary tract during filling and voiding.

External (condom) catheters. Devices for externally draining the bladder made from latex rubber, polyvinyl, or silicone that are secured on the shaft of the penis by some form of adhesive and are connected to urine collecting bags by a tube.

Habit training. A behavioral technique that calls for scheduled toileting at regular intervals on a planned basis. Unlike bladder training, there is no systematic effort to motivate the patient to delay voiding and resist urge.

Hydronephrosis. Dilation of the renal pelvis and calices, and sometimes, collecting ducts, secondary to obstruction of urine flow by calculi, tumors, neurologic disorders, or any various congenital anomalies.

Hypermobility of bladder neck. A condition characterized by the descent and displacement of the urethra and bladder neck from their normal anatomic position during physical exertion, usually resulting in leakage of urine. This condition is the most common cause of stress urinary incontinence. Various surgical procedures can be employed to treat this condition (see bladder suspension).

Hyperreflexia. Any exaggeration of reflexes. In urinary incontinence, an involuntary detrusor contraction resulting from a neurologic disorder.

Indwelling catheters. Tube devices inserted into the bladder, urinary reservoir, or urinary conduit for a period of time longer than one emptying.

Intermittent catheterization. The use of catheters inserted through the urethra into the bladder every 3–6 hours for bladder drainage in persons with urinary retention.

Intrinsic sphincter deficiency (ISD). A cause of stress urinary incontinence in which the urethral sphincter is unable to contract and generate sufficient resistance in the bladder, especially during stress maneuvers. ISD may be due to congenital sphincter weakness, such as myelomeningocele or epispadias, or it may be acquired subsequent to prostatectomy, trauma, radiation therapy, or sacral cord lesions.

Involuntary detrusor contraction. A cause of urinary incontinence resulting from uncontrolled contractions of the detrusor.

Mixed urinary incontinence. The combination, in a patient, of urge urinary incontinence and stress urinary incontinence (see urge incontinence, stress incontinence).

Nocturnal enuresis. The involuntary loss of urine (urinary incontinence) during sleep. Also called bed-wetting.

Overactive bladder. A condition characterized by involuntary detrusor contractions during the bladder filling phase, which may be spontaneous or provoked and which the patient cannot suppress.

Overflow incontinence. The involuntary loss of urine associated with overdistension of the bladder. Overflow incontinence results from urinary retention that causes the capacity of the bladder to be overwhelmed. Continuous or intermittent leakage of a small amount of urine results.

Pelvic muscle exercises (PMEs). A behavioral technique that requires repetitive active exercise of the pubococcygeus muscle to improve urethral resistance and urinary control by strengthening the periurethral and pelvic muscles. Also called Kegel exercises or pelvic floor exercises.

Periurethral bulking injections. A surgical treatment for urethral sphincter insufficiency that involves injecting materials such as polytetrafluoroethylene (PTFE) or collagen into the periurethral area to increase urethral compression.

Pessaries. Devices for women that are placed intravaginally to treat pelvic relaxation or prolapse of pelvic organs.

Pharmacologic treatment. The use of medications to treat urinary incontinence.

Post-void residual (PVR) volume. The amount of fluid remaining in the bladder immediately following the completion of urination. Estimation of PVR volume can be made by abdominal palpation and percussion or bimanual examination. Specific measurement of PVR volume can be accomplished by catheterization, pelvic ultrasound, radiography, or radioisotope studies.

Prompted voiding. A behavioral technique for use primarily with dependent or cognitively impaired persons. Prompted voiding attempts to teach the incontinent person awareness of his/her incontinence status and to request toileting assistance, either independently or after being prompted by a caregiver.

Sensory urgency. Urgency associated with bladder hypersensitivity (see urge/urgency).

Sling procedures. Surgical methods for treating urinary incontinence involving the placement of a sling, made either of tissue obtained from the person undergoing the sling procedure or of tissue obtained from another source, under the urethrovesical junction and anchored to retropubic and/or abdominal structures.

Stress urinary incontinence. A form of urinary incontinence characterized by the involuntary loss of urine from the urethra during physical exertion; for example, during coughing. The stress incontinence symptom or complaint may be confirmed by observing urine loss coincident with an increase in abdominal pressure in the absence of a detrusor contraction or an overdistended bladder (see hypermobility of bladder neck and intrinsic sphincter deficiency).

Suprapubic cystostomy. A surgical procedure involving insertion of a tube or similar instrument through the anterior abdominal wall above the symphysis pubis into the bladder to permit urine drainage from the bladder.

Transient urinary incontinence. Temporary episodes of urinary incontinence that are reversible once the cause or causes of the episode(s) are identified and treated.

Ultrasonography. A technique that uses ultrasound to obtain visual images of the urinary tract for the purpose of assessing its anatomic status.

Underactive bladder. A condition characterized by a bladder contraction of inadequate magnitude and/or duration to effect bladder emptying in a normal timespan. This condition can be caused by drugs, fecal impaction, and neurologic conditions such as diabetic neuropathy or low spinal cord injury or as a result of radical pelvic surgery. It also can result from a weakening of the detrusor muscle from vitamin B_{12} deficiency or idiopathic causes. Bladder underactivity may cause overdistension of the bladder, resulting in overflow incontinence (see overflow incontinence).

Urethral pressure profilometry (UPP). A technique used to measure resting and dynamic pressures in the urethra.

Urethral sphincter mechanism. The segment of the urethra that influences storage and emptying of urine in the bladder. It controls bladder voiding by relaxing, which opens the outlet from the bladder, allowing urine to flow from the bladder to the outside of the body. A deficiency of the urethral sphincter mechanism may allow leakage of urine in the absence of a detrusor contraction.

Urge incontinence. The involuntary loss of urine associated with an abrupt and strong desire to void (urgency). Urge incontinence is usually associated with the urodynamic findings of involuntary detrusor contractions or detrusor overactivity (see detrusor external sphincter dyssynergia, detrusor hyperactivity with impaired bladder contractility, detrusor instability, hyperreflexia, sensory urgency).

Urge/urgency. A strong desire to void.

Urinary incontinence (UI). Involuntary loss of urine sufficient to be a problem. There are several types of UI, but all are characterized by an inability to restrain or control urinary voiding (see mixed urinary incontinence, nocturnal enuresis, overflow incontinence, stress incontinence, transient urinary incontinence, urge incontinence).

Urinary tract. Passageway from the pelvis of the kidney to the urinary orifice through the ureters, bladder, and urethra.

Urinary tract infection (UTI). An infection in the urinary tract caused by the invasion of disease-causing micro-organisms, which proceed to establish themselves, multiply, and produce various symptoms in their host. Infection of the bladder, better known as cystitis, is particularly common in women, mainly because of the much shorter urethra, which provides less of a barrier to bacteria. In men, infection is usually associated with obstruction to the flow of urine, such as prostate gland enlargement.

Urodynamic tests. Tests designed to determine the anatomic and functional status of the urinary bladder and urethra (see cystometry, electromyography, urethral pressure profilometry, uroflowmetry, videourodynamics).

Uroflowmetry. A urodynamic test that measures urine flow either visually, electronically, or with the use of a disposable flowmeter unit.

Vesicoureteric reflux. Backflow of urine from the bladder into the ureter, unilaterally or bilaterally, during rest or especially during urination. The condition may be congenital, secondary to obstruction of the urinary outflow tract, or any disease involving the urinary ureteral orifices.

Videourodynamics. A technique that combines the various urodynamic tests with simultaneous fluoroscopy. Fluoroscopy is a technique for examining internal structures by viewing the shadows cast on a fluorescent screen by objects or parts through which x-rays are directed.

Voiding or bladder diary (record). Also called an "incontinence chart." A record maintained by the patient or caregiver that is used to record the frequency, timing, amount of voiding, and/or other factors associated with the patient's urinary incontinence.

Contributors

Urinary Incontinence in Adults Guideline Update Panel

J. Andrew Fantl, MD, *Co-Chair*
Professor and Vice Chairman
Department of Obstetrics, Gynecology and Reproductive Medicine
Division of Gynecology and General Obstetrics
State University of New York at Stony Brook
Stony Brook, New York
Specialty: Obstetrics/Gynecology
Dr. Fantl served for 20 years as professor in the Department of Obstetrics and
Gynecology before assuming his present position. Dr. Fantl is past president of
the American Urogynecologic Society and the Society of Gynecologic Surgeons.
He currently serves on advisory groups to the International Continence Society
and Help for Incontinent People. His research interests have been urinary incontinence and pelvic organ prolapse in women, areas in which he has published for
the past 15 years. He has been the principal investigator of NIH-NIA funded collaborative research on urinary incontinence and has patented a sensor catheter in
collaboration with the National Aeronautics and Space Administration.

Diane Kaschak Newman, RNC, MSN, FAAN, *Co-Chair*
Adult Nurse Practitioner
Access to Continence Care & Treatment, Inc.
Philadelphia, Pennsylvania
Specialty: Nursing
Ms. Newman is an adult nurse practitioner, consultant, educator, and international speaker specializing in the areas of urinary incontinence and the management
of incontinence. She holds a Master's degree in Nursing from the University of
Pennsylvania. Her private practice, DKN & Associates and Golden Horizons,
provides evaluation and treatment in office practice, long-term care settings for
adult patients, and home care services for incontinent clients. Ms. Newman is
founder and President of Access to Continence Care & Treatment, Inc., an organization that actively promotes the development of incontinence services and
produces educational materials on incontinence for health care providers. Ms.
Newman participated in the University of Pennsylvania School of Nursing
Urinary Incontinence Project in 1986 and was involved with several research
projects on the effect of behavioral treatment for urinary incontinence. She was a
nurse practitioner consultant to the VNA of Trenton/Robert Wood Johnson
Foundation demonstration project, Urinary Incontinence in a Visiting Nursing
Agency. Ms. Newman is a clinical faculty preceptor in the geriatric and adult
nurse practitioner programs at the University of Pennsylvania School of Graduate
Nursing and was chair of the Second National Multi-Specialty Nursing

Conference on Urinary Continence held in January 1994. Ms. Newman has presented scientific papers at national and international meetings, written journal articles, and contributed chapters to publications on the subject of incontinence. She is the editor of the geriatric nursing textbook, *Geriatric Care Plans*.

Joyce Colling, PhD, RN, FAAN
Professor and Chairperson
Community Health Care Systems Department
School of Nursing
Oregon Health Sciences University
Portland, Oregon
Specialty: Nursing

Dr. Colling is a nurse and professor specializing in issues of gerontology. She has contributed much to research on incontinence in the frail elderly in the community and particularly in long-term care settings, with emphasis on staff education to improve incontinence care, and has published numerous research articles on incontinence in the elderly. She provides continence services to clinic patients and consultation to nursing home and community agencies. She is a fellow of the American Academy of Nursing and the Gerontological Society of America and currently serves on two international panels on urinary incontinence.

John O.L. DeLancey, MD
Associate Professor and Director of Gynecology
Department of Obstetrics and Gynecology
University of Michigan Medical Center
Ann Arbor, Michigan
Specialty: Obstetrics/Gynecology

Dr. DeLancey's area of research focuses on understanding the pathophysiology of urinary incontinence and problems with pelvic organ support. His clinical practice centers around surgical management of urinary incontinence and pelvic organ prolapse. He is president-elect of the American Urogynecologic Society and has lectured extensively in the United States and abroad concerning urinary incontinence.

Christopher Keeys, PharmD
President
Clinical Pharmacy Associates
Calverton, Maryland
Specialty: Pharmacy

Dr. Keeys is presently co-founder and president of Clinical Pharmacy Associates, Inc. He received his Bachelor of Science degree, magna cum laude, from Howard University in 1980 and his Doctor of Pharmacy degree in 1982 from the Philadelphia College of Pharmacy and Sciences. He is a registered pharmacist in Washington, DC, Maryland, Virginia, and Pennsylvania. During the past 15 years of professional life he has provided, through innovation and team building, progressive pharmaceutical services for many health care organizations, and served as a teacher of students and colleagues. His works and writings on the subjects of drug information, adverse drug reactions, and contemporary pharmacy practice have been published in professional and public press both in the United States and abroad. He has been active in local and national professional organizations and is currently serving as Chairman, Drug Use Review Board, District of Columbia, and Co-Vice Chairman, Chesapeake Research Review, Inc., an ethical research committee. Dr. Keeys has been honored as the recipient of the Honored Preceptor Award from the Doctor of Pharmacy Class, Howard University; Pharmacist of the Year award from the Washington Metropolitan Society of Hospital Pharmacists; and Distinguished Pharmacy Alumnus Award from the Howard University Pharmacy Alumnus Association.

Richard M. Loughery, FACHA
Planning Consultant
National Museum of Health and Medicine
McLean, Virginia
Specialty: Hospital Administration, Consumer Representative
Mr. Loughery served as special assistant and director of the Advisory Committee Office of the Secretary of the Department of Health and Human Services, Public Health Service. In this position, he advised the Secretary about a variety of health care and policy issues. For over 20 years he was the chief executive officer and president of the Washington Hospital Center, a 910-bed teaching hospital. He has served in leadership positions with the American Hospital Association and the American College of Hospital Administrators.

B. Joan McDowell, PhD, CRNP, FAAN
Associate Professor of Nursing
University of Pittsburgh
Pittsburgh, Pennsylvania
Specialty: Nursing
Dr. McDowell received her doctorate in Higher Education Administration at the University of Pittsburgh. Since 1981, she has been affiliated with the University of Pittsburgh School of Medicine, where she serves as associate professor of nursing, director of the continence program, and assistant research professor of medicine. Dr. McDowell is a Fellow in the American Academy of Nursing and the recipient of many awards, including the Pennsylvania Nurses Associa-tion Commonwealth Award for Nursing Practice, the Award of Excellence from the American Academy of Nurse Practitioners, and inclusion in Who's Who in American Nursing. She has been the principal investigator for the Behavioral Treatment of Urinary Incontinence in Homebound Elderly since 1992, and during that time has authored and coauthored several articles on the identification and treatment of urinary incontinence.

Peggy A. Norton, MD
Associate Professor
Department of Obstetrics and Gynecology
University of Utah School of Medicine
Salt Lake City, Utah
Specialty: Obstetrics/Gynecology

Dr. Norton is a gynecologist specializing in urodynamics and surgery for urinary incontinence and genital prolapse. She has published numerous papers on these two subjects, and has co-authored three textbooks on urinary incontinence. She is principal investigator on an NIH-funded study on the role of connective tissue in genitourinary prolapse. She is currently the research chairman for the American Urogynecologic Society and serves on several national and international advisory panels for the NIH, Society of Gynecologic Surgeons, and the International Continence Society. She recently won a teaching award from the American College of Obstetricians and Gynecologists.

Joseph Ouslander, MD
Vice President, Medical Affairs
Jewish Home for the Aging
Associate Professor
Multicampus Division of Geriatric Medicine and Gerontology
UCLA School of Medicine
Reseda, California
Specialty: Geriatrics

Dr. Ouslander is associate professor of medicine in the Multicampus Division of Geriatric Medicine and Gerontology at the University of California, Los Angeles School of Medicine, associate director of the Borun Center for Gerontological Research, and director of Gerontology at Encino Hospital. Dr. Ouslander has served on several national and international panels on urinary incontinence, has published numerous research articles on incontinence and has coauthored two books. He currently serves on the Board of Directors of the American Geriatrics Society and has served on the Geriatric Medicine Test Committee of the American Board of Internal Medicine/American Board of Family Practice.

John F. Schnelle, PhD
Director and Professor-in-Residence
Borun Center for Gerontological Research
UCLA School of Medicine and Jewish Home for the Aging
Reseda, California
Specialty: Psychology, Gerontology

Dr. Schnelle is director of the Borun Center for Gerontological Research and a professor at the Multicampus Division of Geriatric Medicine and Gerontology, School of Medicine, University of California, Los Angeles. He is known for his role as principal investigator on several major clinical trial intervention grants designed to improve care and management in nursing homes and has received awards for his outstanding contributions to behavior therapy. Among his most notable contributions is his innovative work in incontinence care, comprehensively described in his book, *Management of Urinary Incontinence in the Frail Elderly*. Dr. Schnelle has published in the areas of quality control in institutional settings and quality of life issues in the frail elderly, with over 100 publications in professional books and journals.

David R. Staskin, MD
Director
Urodynamics and Incontinence Center
Harvard Medical School
Beth Israel Hospital
Boston, Massachusetts
Specialty: Urology
Dr. Staskin is an assistant professor of surgery/urology at Harvard Medical School and Director of the Urodynamics and Continence Center at Beth Israel Hospital in Boston, where he holds teaching positions in both the divisions of Urology and Gynecology. He is also the Chief of Surgery at Malden Hospital. He currently serves on the Outcome Measures Committee for the International Continence Society, the Board of Directors of the American Urogynecologic Society and the Massachusetts Multiple Sclerosis Association, and is a member of the Urodynamics Society of the American Urological Association. His research and clinical interests are concentrated in the evaluation and treatment of incontinence and voiding dysfunction.

Jeannette M. Tries, MS, OTR
Director
Biofeedback and Incontinence Centers
Sacred Heart Rehabilitation Hospital
Milwaukee, Wisconsin
Specialty: Occupational Therapy, Psychology
Ms. Tries is president of the Clinic for Neurological Learning and is a consultant to the University of Illinois Incontinence Service within the Colon-Rectal Surgery Department. A registered occupational therapist and certified biofeedback therapist, Ms. Tries has developed neuromuscular reeducation and incontinencebiofeedback programs. She is past president of the Biofeedback Society of Wisconsin, past board member of the Biofeedback Certification Institute of America, as well as consultant to faculties developing electromyographic neuromuscular reeducation and incontinence programs. Ms. Tries has a strong interest in development of behavioral and reeducation strategies for the neurologically impaired.

Vernon C. Urich, MD
Chief
Urology Section and Urodynamic Lab
Carl T. Hayden VA Medical Center
Phoenix, Arizona
Specialty: Urology
Dr. Urich is a urologist, surgeon, and educator, whose main interest is patient education. He was president of the Michigan Urological Society in 1990 and was on that Society's Board of Directors for 5 years. He is currently on the editorial board of *Patient Education and Counseling* and formerly was on the board of directors of the International Patient Education Council and the board of trustees of the Center for Gerontology. He was a member of the Urinary Incontinence Guideline Panel and now serves on the VA Institute of Quality Management Guideline Panel. Prior to recent relocation, he was on the faculty of the University of Michigan and Michigan State University.

Sharon H. Vitousek, MD
Waimea Medical Associates
Lucy Henriques Medical Center
Kamuela, Hawaii
Specialty: Primary Care, Community Health
Dr. Vitousek received her medical degree from the John Burns School of Medicine in Hawaii. Currently, she is president of the State of Hawaii Board of Health, and maintains a part-time internal medicine practice with Waimea Medical Associates. She has also worked as a clinical professor of medicine for Queen Emma Clinic.   Dr. Vitousek has long been involved in community efforts to improve the health status of individuals in North Hawaii. She wrote the mission statement for North Hawaii Community Hospital, Inc., worked with the Department of Health to develop a public/private partnership for its funding, developed a proposal to procure a $2 million grant for the hospital, and served as its president. In 1994, Dr. Vitousek was elected to the Hawaii Medical Association House of Delegates.

Barry D. Weiss, MD
Professor of Family Medicine
Department of Family and Community Medicine
University of Arizona
College of Medicine
Tucson, Arizona
Specialty: Family Medicine, Geriatrics
Dr. Weiss serves on national committees of the American Academy of Family Physicians, the National Cancer Institute, and the Agency for Health Care Policy and Research. He is editor of *Family Medicine*, the national journal of the Society of Teachers of Family Medicine. Dr. Weiss is the author of over 80 publications in peer-reviewed medical journals, and serves on the

Arizona Board of Medical Examiners, the regulatory agency responsible for licensing and disciplining physicians who practice medicine in Arizona.

Kristene Whitmore, MD
Chief of Urology, Director of the Incontinence Center
The Graduate Hospital
Philadelphia, Pennsylvania
Specialty: Urology
Dr. Whitmore, in addition to her responsibilities at The Graduate Hospital, also serves on the urology staff for the Philadelphia Veteran's Administration Hospital and is a clinical professor of urology at the University of Pennsylvania. Over the past 16 years, Dr. Whitmore has presented nationally and internationally and has authored or coauthored more than 100 articles and books. Dr. Whitmore has made numerous television appearances, and served for 3 years as a medical consultant for the Emmy award-winning drama, "St. Elsewhere." She has also provided consultation to Searle, Merck, Sharp and Dohme, Marion, Johnson & Johnson, and Wang laboratories. Dr. Whitmore is a member of the American Medical Association, American Association of Clinical Urologists, American Urogynecological Society, American Foundation for Urologic Diseases, National Kidney Foundation, and International Continence Society. She was the 1994 president of Women in Urology and was listed in *Who's Who Worldwide*.

Consultants

Patricia Burns, PhD, RN, FAAN
Director, School of Nursing
Department of Graduate Education
SUNY of Buffalo
Buffalo, New York

Ananias Diokno, MD
Chief, Department of Urology
William Beaumont Hospital
Royal Oak, Michigan

Teh-Wei Hu, PhD
Professor of Health Economics
Department of Social and
   Administrative Health Sciences
Berkeley, California

Donna Katzman McClish, PhD
Associate Professor
Department of Biostatistics
Medical College of Virginia
Richmond, Virginia

**Thelma Joan Wells, PhD, RN,
FAAN**
University of Wisconsin
   School of Nursing
Madison, Wisconsin

Matthew Zack, MD, MPH
Centers for Disease Control
   and Prevention
Atlanta, Georgia

AHCPR Staff

Douglas B. Kamerow, MD, MPH
*Director, Office of the Forum for
   Quality and Effectiveness
   in Health Care*

Francis Chesley, MD
Senior Health Policy Analyst

Margaret Coopey, MGA, RN
Senior Health Policy Analyst

Stan Edinger, MD
Senior Health Policy Analyst

Carole Hudgings, PhD
Senior Health Policy Analyst

Lawrence C. McMurtry, MSSW
Senior Health Policy Analyst

Randie A. Siegel
Senior Health Policy Analyst

Karen N. Carp
Public Affairs Specialist

Contract Support

Technical Resources International, Inc.
   Rockville, Maryland

Gail J. Herzenberg, MPA
Project Director

Cheryl Campbell
Panel Manager

Marcia R. Feinleib
Managing Editor

Joan A. Saunders
Panel Editor

Joanna Taylor
Production Editor

David Tran
Literature Acquisition Specialist

John Warner, MS
Research Analyst

Peer Reviewers[a]

Anne Alberg
Vice President, Sales and Marketing
Diagnostic Ultrasound Corporation
Redmond, Washington

Margaret M. Baumann, MD
Section of Geriatric Medicine
University of Illinois at Chicago
Chicago, Illinois

Kari Bo, PE, PT, PhD
Associate Professor
The Norwegian University of Sport
  and Physical Education
Oslo, Norway

Carol Brink, MPH, RN
Associate Professor of
  Clinical Nursing
University of Rochester
  School of Nursing
Rochester, New York

Norman Bruckner, PhD
Director, Product Development
Johnson & Johnson
Arlington, Texas

Richard Bump, MD
Associate Professor
Department of
  Obstetrics/Gynecology
Duke University
Durham, North Carolina

Kathryn Burgio, PhD
Associate Professor of Medicine
Division of Gerontology and
  Geriatric Medicine
University of Alabama
Birmingham, Alabama

Amanda Clark, MD
Oregon Health Sciences University
Portland, Oregon

Dr. Alan Cottenden
Lecturer
Department of Medical Physics
  and Bioengineering
University College London
London, England

Molly Dougherty, PhD, RN
Professor and Research Coordinator
University of Florida College
  of Nursing
Gainesville, Florida

Carol Einhorn, RN
Gerontological Nurse Practitioner
VA West Side Medical Center
Chicago, Illinois

Sheila Fiers, RN, BSN, CETN
Rochester, Minnesota

Norman F. Gant, MD
Executive Director
American Board of
  Obstetrics/Gynecology
Dallas, Texas

Mikel Gray
Department of Urology
University of Virginia Health
  Sciences Center
Charlottesville, Virginia

Constance Halverson, RN
Clinical Research Advisor
EMPI, Inc.
Minneapolis, Minnesota

---

[a] These individuals provided peer review. Their participation does not necessarily imply endorsement of the guideline.

Kay E. Jewell, MD
Health Care Financing
Administration
Baltimore, Maryland

Aaron Kirkemo, MD
Director, Urodynamics Laboratory
Henry Ford Hospital
Detroit, Michigan

Beverly Korfin, RN
Urologic Division
CR Bard, Inc.
Covington, Georgia

Rhonda Kotarinos, MS, PT
President
Women's Therapeutic Services, Ltd.
Chicago, Illinois

Gary Leach, MD
Department of Urology
Kaiser Permanente Medical Center
Los Angeles, California

Deborah Lekan-Rutledge, MSN
University of North Carolina,
 Chapel Hill
Chapel Hill, North Carolina

Edward McGuire, MD
Professor and Director
Division of Urology
University of Texas-Houston
Houston, Texas

Mark McIntyre
American Medical Systems
Minneapolis, Minnesota

Joseph Montella, MD
Assistant Professor
Department of Obstetrics
 and Gynecology
Jefferson Medical College
Philadelphia, Pennsylvania

Julie Graves Moy, MD
American Academy of Family
 Physicians
Houston, Texas

Christine Norton, MA, RN
Director
The Continence Foundation
London, England

Mary Palmer, RNC, PhD
Senior Staff Fellow
National Institute of
 Nursing Research
National Institutes of Health
Baltimore, Maryland

Richard Reed, MD
Director, Geriatric Programs
University of Minnesota
 Medical School
Minneapolis, Minnesota

Patricia Rowell, RN
American Nurses Association
Washington, DC

Carolyn Sampselle, PhD, RN
Associate Professor
University of Michigan
School of Nursing
Ann Arbor, Michigan

Dr. Kathleen Siegwart
Personal Products
Johnson & Johnson
Dayton, New Jersey

Stuart Smythe
Vice President
Laborie Medical Technologies
 Corporation
South Burlington, Vermont

Christopher Steidle, MD
Urologist
Northeast Indiana Urology, PC
Fort Wayne, Indiana

Morton A. Stenchever, MD
Professor and Chairman
Department of Obstetrics &
  Gynecology
University of Washington
  School of Medicine
Seattle, Washington

Jim Stupar
Incare Medical Products
Libertyville, Illinois

Kathe Wallace, PT
Northlake Physical Therapy
Seattle, Washington

John Warren, MD
Head, Division of Infectious
  Diseases
University of Maryland
  School of Medicine
Baltimore, Maryland

Adeline Yerkes, MPH
Chief, Chronic Disease Services
Oklahoma State Department
  of Health
Oklahoma City, Oklahoma

Attachments

Attachment A. Management of Urinary Incontinence in Primary Care

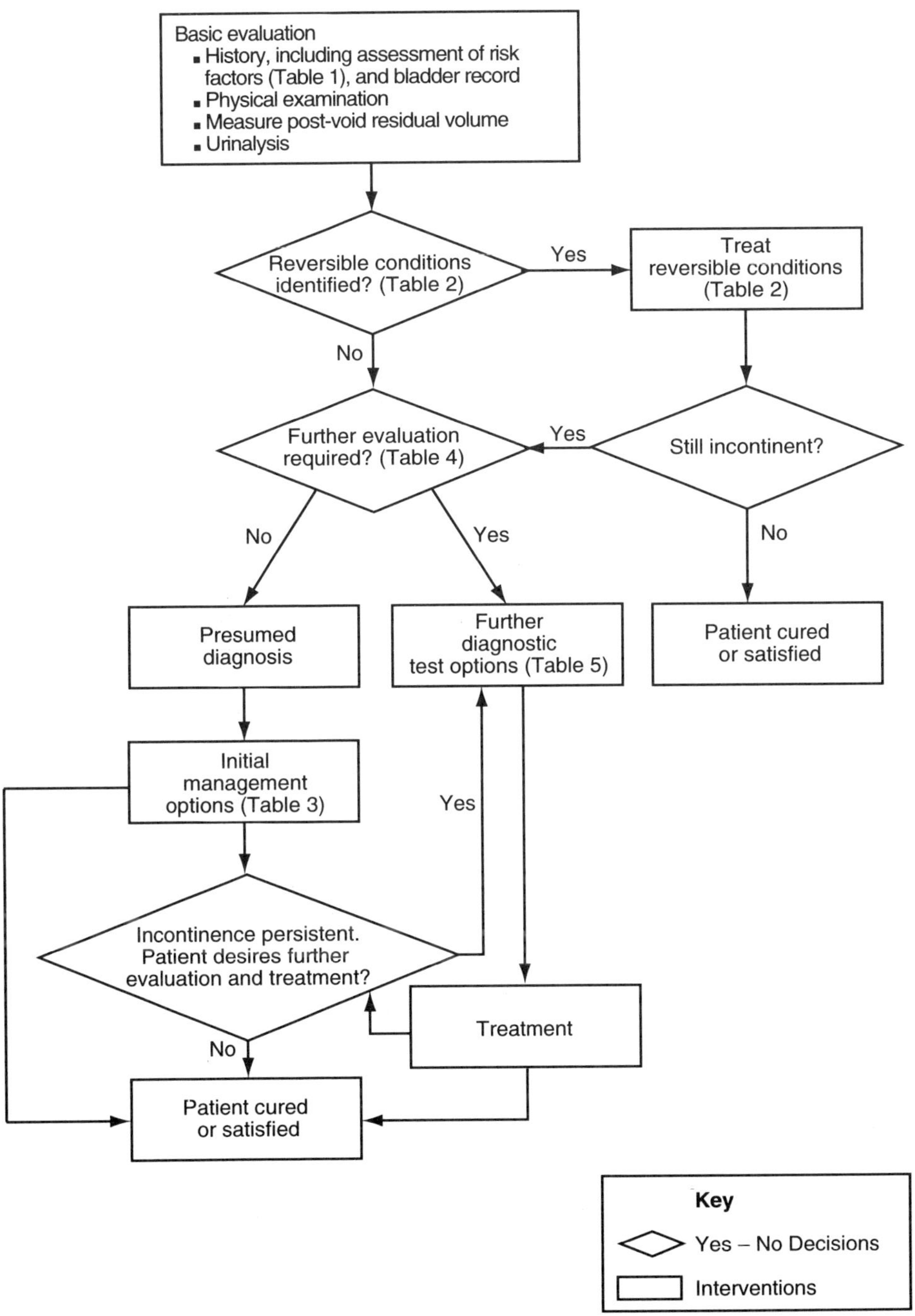

Attachment B. Sample Bladder Record

NAME: ____

DATE: ____

INSTRUCTIONS: Place a check in the appropriate column next to the time you urinated in the toilet or when an incontinence episode occurred. Note the reason for the incontinence and describe your liquid intake (for example, coffee, water) and estimate the amount (for example, one cup).

Time interval	Urinated in toilet	Had a small incontinence episode	Had a large incontinence episode	Reason for incontinence episode	Type/amount of liquid intake
6–8 a.m.					
8–10 a.m.					
10–noon					
Noon–2 p.m.					
2–4 p.m.					
4–6 p.m.					
6–8 p.m.					
8–10 p.m.					
10–midnight					
Overnight					

No. of pads used today: _______________ No. of episodes: _______________

Comments: ____

____

____

Attachment C. Sample Incontinence Monitoring Record for Hospital and Nursing Home Patients

INSTRUCTIONS: EACH TIME THE PATIENT IS CHECKED:
1) Mark one of the circles in the BLADDER section at the hour closest to the time the patient is checked.
2) Make an X in the BOWEL section if the patient has had an incontinent or normal bowel movement.

| ✔ = Incontinent, small amount | ⌀ = Dry | × = Incontinence BOWEL |
| ✔ = Incontinent, large amount | N = Voided correctly | × = Normal BOWEL |

PATIENT NAME _______________________________ ROOM # _____ DATE __________

TIME	BLADDER			BOWEL			
	Incontinence of urine	Dry	Voided correctly	Incontinence	Normal	Initials	Comments
12 am	• •	○	Δ cc _______				
1	• •	○	Δ cc _______				
2	• •	○	Δ cc _______				
3	• •	○	Λ cc _______				
4	• •	○	Δ cc _______				
5	• •	○	Δ cc _______				
6	• •	○	Δ cc _______				
7	• •	○	Δ cc _______				
8	• •	○	Δ cc _______				
9	• •	○	Δ cc _______				
10	• •	○	Δ cc _______				
11	• •	○	Δ cc _______				
12 pm	• •	○	Δ cc _______				
1	• •	○	Δ cc _______				
2	• •	○	Δ cc _______				
3	• •	○	Δ cc _______				
4	• •	○	Δ cc _______				
5	• •	○	Δ cc _______				
6	• •	○	Δ cc _______				
7	• •	○	Δ cc _______				
8	• •	○	Δ cc _______				
9	• •	○	Δ cc _______				
10	• •	○	Δ cc _______				
11	• •	○	Δ cc _______				
TOTALS:							

Index

Tricyclic antidepressants or agents, 44, 46

U

Ultrasonography, 30
Unconscious incontinence.
See Reflex incontinence
Unstable bladder, 44, 69
Upper tract imaging, 29
Urethral diverticulum, 24
Urethral hypermobility, 24, 52, 54
Urethral pressure profilometry (UPP), 26, 28
Urethral sphincter insufficiency, 16, 48–49
Urethrolysis, 64
Urethritis, 14, 68

Urge incontinence, 13, 25–26, 39, 43–44
Urinalysis, 22, 53
Urinary tract infection (UTI), 14, 58
Urine cytology, 23
Urodynamic tests, 27, 55
Uroflowmetry, 26, 28

V

Vaginal weight training, 36, 41
Vaginitis, 72–73. *See also* Atrophic vaginitis
Valsalva leak point, 53
Vesicoureteral reflux, 13, 18, 30, 62, 65
Videourodynamics, 26, 30

X

Xerostomia, 45, 47, 49

Notes

Notes